HEALTHY
EXERCISE
HABITS

HEALTHY EXERCISE HABITS

From Planning ➔ to Action ➔ to Results

A HEALTHY HABITS SYSTEM

LAURA SARTI

Visit author's website to learn more at www.AndiamoFit.com

Disclaimer All content in this material is created for educational and informational purposes only. The information is not intended or implied to be a substitute for professional medical advice, diagnosis or treatment. It does not take into account your individual health, medical, physical or emotional situation or needs. It is not a substitute for medical attention, treatment, examination, advice, treatment of existing conditions or diagnosis and is not intended to provide a clinical diagnosis nor take the place of proper medical advice from a fully qualified medical practitioner. You should, before you act or use any of this information, consider the appropriateness of this information having regard to your own personal situation and needs. You are responsible for consulting a suitable medical professional and/or exercise specialist before using any of the information or materials contained in our material or accessed through our website, before trying any treatment or taking any course of action that may directly or indirectly affect your health or well-being. The author makes no representation and assumes no responsibility for the accuracy of information contained in or available in this book, and such information is subject to change without notice. You are encouraged to confirm any information obtained from or through this book with other sources, and review all information regarding any medical condition or treatment with your physician.

Always seek the guidance of your doctor or other qualified health professional with any questions you may have regarding your health or a medical condition. Never disregard the advice of a medical professional, or delay in seeking it because of something you have read in this book.

Always consult your physician before beginning any exercise program. This general information is not intended to diagnose any medical condition or to replace your healthcare professional. Consult with your healthcare professional to design an appropriate exercise prescription. If you experience any pain or difficulty with these exercises, stop and consult your healthcare provider.

This disclaimer states that there is no guarantee of specific results and individual results may vary. We cannot and do not guarantee that you will attain a specific or particular result, and you accept the risk that results differ for each individual. The health and fitness success depends on each individual's background, dedication, desire, and motivation. As with any health-related program or service, your results may vary, and will be based on many variables, including but not limited to, your individual capacity, life experience, unique health and genetic profile, starting point, expertise, and level of commitment.

We expressly disclaim responsibility to any person or entity for any liability, loss, or damage caused or alleged to be caused directly or indirectly as a result of the use, application or interpretation of any material provided.

WHEN TO CONTACT YOUR PHYSICIAN

If you experience any symptoms of weakness, unsteadiness, light-headedness or dizziness, chest pain or pressure, nausea, or shortness of breath. Mild soreness after exercise may be experienced after beginning a new exercise. Contact your physician if the soreness does not improve after 2-3 days.

If you think you may have a medical emergency, call your doctor, go to the nearest hospital emergency department, or call the emergency services immediately. If you choose to rely on any information provided by this book you do so solely at your own risk.

Book Design by Reider Books. Book Cover Design by ebooklaunch.com. Images by Pixabay

For our past selves, my inspiration for writing this book, forgiven for trying our best but not always succeeding. For our future selves, may we join together to age gracefully, to look forward to a future bright with possibilities, one small step at a time.

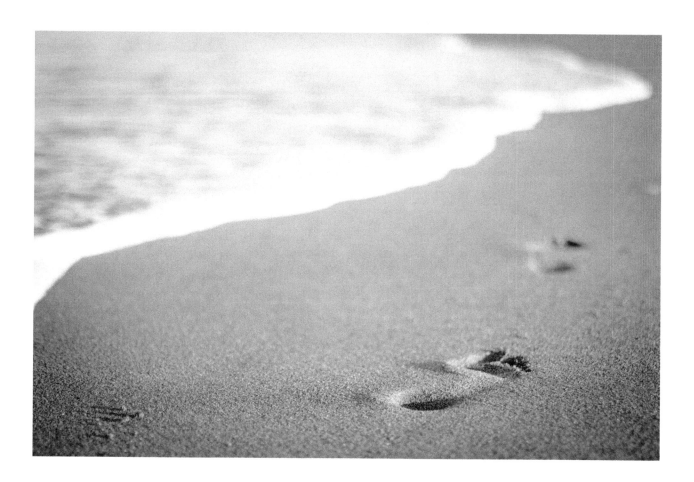

TABLE OF CONTENTS

PREFACE

Hi! My name is Laura, and I am a registered nurse, a certified health coach, certified personal trainer, and founder of AndiamoFit. I have a bachelor's degree in nursing, a bachelor's degree in sociology, and a master's degree in teaching. And I've been studying motivation and behavioral change for years.

I developed a healthy exercise habits *system* because I am on a personal mission to help people live their best lives, by taking them on a journey of small steps and simple sustainable habits. I am doing this because I know the value of exercise in helping prevent lifestyle disease. I've seen what happens to people when lifestyle diseases hit them hard. *And I would not wish this on anyone.* My goal is to ease suffering and to do my part to help people restore their health.

But I also know how hard it can be to *just start*. And I know that it can be even harder to just *stick with something*. Our days can be loud, busy, hectic, and often times chaotic, leaving us feeling drained and with little energy leftover to make healthy changes. Being healthy requires a shift in our collective paradigm, and I want to help make that shift happen. Being healthy in today's world requires a bit of effort. It requires a *decision* to make your health a priority. It also requires awareness, mindfulness, and a *plan*.

I am here for you, and I want to do this together, *with* you. With a little bit of self-awareness, a solid plan in place, and by answering the right questions, we can do this in a way that is simple, safe, and will only require a series of small easy steps. So let *this* be your guide toward getting moving again, one small step at a time. Because we already know that if you don't move it, you lose it!

INTRODUCTION

Almost fifty years ago, a colleague of my dad's told him that maybe he should try jogging. He told him that it was a good habit to adopt and that he might like it. Very soon after this seemingly simple yet life-altering suggestion, something in my dad's mind just shifted. One day he woke up and he started jogging. Just like that. I'm not even sure he had a pair of running shoes when he started!

Since that day, my dad hasn't stopped running. It appeared that my dad's identity changed overnight. He went from someone who didn't exercise at all to someone who was a *jogger*. He is seventy years old now, and this unbreakable morning habit still runs strong. Travel, harsh weather, even illness...nothing stops him from going on his morning jog.

But change does not come as easily for the rest of us mere mortals. On the other side of the family, you have my mom and me—two people who did everything in their power to get out of gym class. I can still recall my seventh-grade gym teacher's reaction after having had the pleasure of witnessing my first gymnastics floor routine. He strongly advised me not to quit my day job (and he was right!). But neither that experience nor any of my other horror stories in gym class (believe me, there were many!) stopped me from embracing exercise later on life.

The Struggle Is Real

We all know that exercise is good for us. We have a million and one apps and novel exercise ideas at our fingertips. We are bombarded with marketing by a booming fitness industry. Yet so many of us still struggle to *just start*.

How many times have you told yourself that you need to exercise more? How many times has someone else in your life tried to encourage you to get moving? If your answer to these questions includes a sigh, an eye roll, and an acknowledgment of familiarity with these statements, then chances are you're in the majority. Less than a quarter of Americans are meeting the current weekly exercise recommendations. This is despite most people knowing the many benefits of exercise.

If exercising regularly were as simple as my dad makes it appear, then you'd already be doing it, right? Then what's stopping you? How do you motivate yourself to get moving and *stay* moving? How can you see the point in daily movement? How do you find the energy and drive to keep at it? How do you go from *knowing* you want to exercise more to *actually* exercising more?

This book answers these questions and many more. By the end of this book, you will have clarity. With this clarity, you will have confidence in yourself. Believe it or not, the answers to these questions are quite simple. There's actually a very good reason that you naturally resist exercise. By reading this book, you will learn what that reason is, as well as ways to work around this. You are going to work *with* your nature, no longer *against* it. You will be able to stick with your goal to exercise more, once and for all. If this is exactly what you want for yourself, then let's begin!

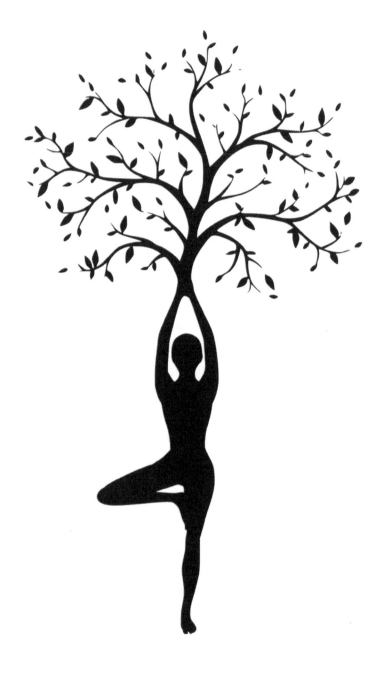

Your Transformation

Envision yourself six months from now. One year from now. Five years from now. What do you *want* to see? The power of visualization is strong. With the right action plan, there is no reason that your visualization cannot become your reality.

You have the ability to transform into a person who's built fitness into your everyday life by completing this workbook. You can learn to appreciate the gift of moving your body. You can learn to appreciate what your body can do. You can do this by keeping an open mind, and you can do this by trusting the *process of change*. With the right mindset, you *can* become a regular and devoted exerciser.

Starting today, I want you to start looking at yourself differently. From now on, identify with who you *want* to become. Stop telling yourself that you're an unfit, unathletic, lazy couch potato. From this moment on, tell yourself that you are strong and capable. Tell yourself that you are an *exerciser*. *Identify* with the change. Tell yourself that you are a person who values health and vitality. You've made other changes in your life, and you've stuck with them before, so there's no reason you can't do it again now.

What This Book *Is*

This book is designed for beginners. It is designed for people who want to be more active and who want to learn how to *create the routine of daily exercise*. This book will introduce a customizable system to introduce the right exercise habits into your life. You will learn more about yourself. You will discover what works for *you*. Therefore, *you* will lead the way. Then, with the personal insights that you obtain, you will learn *how to* successfully make this change. This book will help you adopt new exercise habits by helping you build a *system* that works.

You will also create your own individualized workout plan. You will have the opportunity to reflect on what's working and what isn't. Self-awareness will be paramount.

What This Book Is Not

Before proceeding, you should also know what this book is *not*. This book will not prescribe any specific exercises, nor will it show you *how to do* any specific exercises. It will not go into much detail about the different types of exercises, but it *will* offer you examples of exercises that you can do to help you get started. This book will not dictate to you what you *must do*, and this workbook should definitely not feel like a chore to work on. This book is also not just another exercise log or exercise planner either.

How To Use This Book

The absolute best way to be successful while using this book is to keep one very important thing in mind: *Motivation follows action*. You may not *feel like* putting in the work sometimes. But make sure you do not fall into this trap. Do not sit around and just wait for motivation to strike. Because oftentimes it will not. Take some steps, no matter how small, and I promise you that you will start feeling more motivated as you go along.

Perhaps that little step you take is just telling yourself that you will do one quick push-up, but that you will do it *every single morning*. Or you'll walk just to the end of the short block and back. No matter how you *feel*, you will always be able to do at least this much, every day. The magic happens as soon you see that once you *start moving*, you will usually end up doing far more than you initially set out to. You will rarely do just that *one* push-up. The trick will be to get yourself to take just that first step. Again, *motivation follows action.*

There are four main parts to this book: Reviewing the Basics, The Warm-Up: Building the Foundation for Change, The Workout: Getting Ready for Action, and Cooldown: Sustaining Change.

This book will only work if you do the work. It is not designed to be a feel-good book about your current state. Because remember, you came here looking for a *change*. You know your current path isn't working for you. For this reason, we have to get into *action* mode early on. This process will require some commitment and perseverance from your end. But don't let this slow you down: By opening this book, you've already taken your first step…don't stop now!

One last thing to keep in mind: If you want this to work, you must make a promise to yourself that this book will not end up in the corner collecting dust with all the others. It is not one of those books. If you want this book to be different, then make it *visible* in your living space. Find that one spot in your home where you know you'll come across it each and every day. Make it *easy* to open. And most importantly, *make* (don't just *find*!) time to open it *every single day*. You *will* have time for this… *because if something is important enough to you, then you <u>will</u> make time for it no matter what.*

Activity

Let's begin by writing an intention statement. Intention statements are like promises that you make to yourself. You are making a promise to yourself to commit to this process because you want to change your life for the better. You want to feel vibrant, and you want to feel more energetic. And this time, you are ready to do this. You are doing this today because you can't afford to wait another day to live the life you deserve.

You can write your intention statement in this workbook, but you can also write it on a separate piece of paper. Either way, place these words somewhere prominent in your living space.

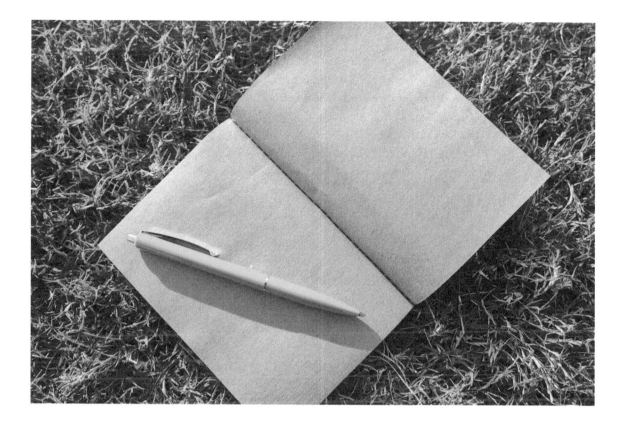

Sample Intention Statement:

"I will open this book every single day for the next <u>30</u> days because I want to lose weight so I can feel strong and confident again."

➢ What can you promise yourself today, as you embark on this new journey of getting healthier?

➢ Who can you share this intention statement with? Is there anyone who would like to join you on this journey?

Okay, great! Now that you've made a commitment to this workbook, we are ready to begin. To get the most out of this experience, it is recommended that you work on this book in the order that it is presented. This is not mandatory, however, and you can skip around if you feel you've already completed some of these steps. But it is highly recommended that you complete each part of the change process in order to make this change stick. Take time to answer the questions truthfully and thoughtfully. You can choose to go at whichever pace is most comfortable for you. As long as you keep moving forward, step by step.

And don't forget ... *any bit of exercise is better than nothing, and it is absolutely never too late to start.* With this in mind, let's begin!

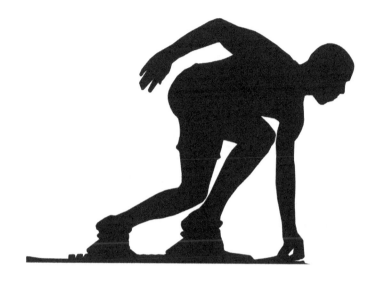

PART ONE

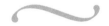

REVIEWING THE BASICS

You are probably reading this book because you are hoping to make your life better in some way. What do you hope to get out of this book? Let's first get clear on this part before proceeding.

To really hype yourself up for change, it is important to review the basics, even if just to remind yourself of the many reasons that this change is a good idea. Any successful change requires first making an informed decision, based on learning the effects that a particular change will have on your life. This really helps prime your mind for change.

Part One will begin by making sure that your head is in the game. Then you are going to discover why it feels so unnatural to exercise just for the sake of exercising. From there, you will be able to continue without feeling guilty about not having *wanted* to exercise in the past. We're going to review what's at stake if you *don't* start exercising, followed by a review of what you can *gain* if you *do* start exercising.

Finally, in Part One, we are going to look at how much exercise is currently recommended and how to get started by learning the most basic fundamental exercise moves. You might be surprised by how basic they really are!

Adopting the Right Mindset

Almost all of the effort that you put into making a change will be made toward shifting your mindset. The how-to and technicalities come later. That's actually the easy part, but it is *not* easy to be motivated to make a change in your life when you're dragging your feet and are barely able to get yourself out of bed in the morning. No amount of motivational videos or fancy fitness apps can get you to do something when your state of mind is not in the right place to begin with. Before confidence, before clarity, and before finding motivation, ask yourself if you are really ready to start living life the way it is meant to be lived. You are here on this earth for but a mere period of time. If you are *truly* living, then it will go by in a flash. Do you really want to spend it by sitting idle and waiting for life to just happen *to* you?

Motivation to make healthy changes can waver when other emotions are not in check, or when either fulfillment or sense of purpose are missing in life. While this is beyond the scope of this book, this is why, when making a healthy change, it can be helpful to consider *all dimensions of wellness.* Taking care of your physical body is only one dimension. Improving *other* aspects of your life can help you spring out of bed every morning, ready to do the things that you know will lead to a better life overall. While you are on this journey, continue to explore other areas of your life that can give you reason to wake up each morning with more vigor. I promise that doing so will allow the habit of daily exercise to come more naturally.

Before proceeding, it would also help to assess your current *attitude* toward exercise. If you are already telling yourself repeatedly, "I hate exercise," then how successful do you think you will be with this change? Your mind has the power to decide which actions you take or don't take. And it all starts with your *attitude*. Rather than tell yourself that you hate all exercise across the board, can you agree that perhaps you just haven't found something that works for you and for your lifestyle? I learned early on in life that gymnastics wasn't for me! But I also discovered certain other exercises that were quite enjoyable. Sure, there are x, y, z reasons to hate exercise. But there are also a multitude of ways to work around this and build exercise into your life once you shift your attitude and make exercise a priority. Are you *willing* to do this?

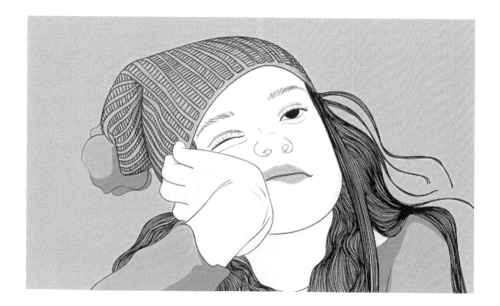

Whenever you notice this sort of negative self-talk that wishes to only keep you in your comfort zone, tell yourself firmly to STOP IT. Tell yourself that you will continue exploring your options, that you *will* make it work this time. If you believe that you want this and you believe that you will change, then you will succeed. If you believe you will fail and you enter into this with a negative attitude, then you will fail. This is totally up to you. Be your own advocate, your own strongest supporter. Because you *can* do this and because you *deserve* this.

Activity

✓ Answer honestly. What is your self-talk about exercise? How do you really feel about it?

✓ If your attitude about exercise is negative, how can you reframe this and shift your perspective to make it more positive?

Example: "I hate exercise" can become "I don't hate *all* exercise. I just haven't found one that I find enjoyable or that works in my life. But I will not give up because I know exercise is important. I will have fun trying new things until I *will* find what works for me."

Getting Rid of the Guilt

From this moment on, I want you to stop blaming yourself. You are going to leave the guilt, the shame, and the labeling at the door. It is *not your fault* that you don't like to exercise. It is not your fault that you often don't see a point in moving your body. To understand why we are naturally "lazy," we must look no further than our wild human ancestors. As with many of life's most pressing questions, the answer lies in nature. We must look at those whose genes we've inherited, the ones who spent their days not in today's society with modern-day amenities, but in the wild where food was often scarce and resources limited. Because the truth is, we aren't wired all that differently from them. And while our ancestors were not lazy, per se, they *were* survivors who made calculated decisions when it came to using up their precious energy.

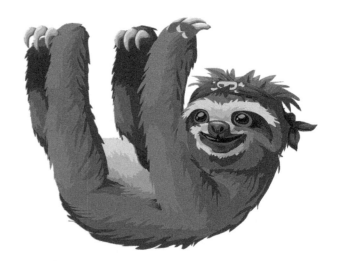

Let me ask you this: In a natural environment when food is scarce, would you say it would be *lazy* or *prudent* to conserve your energy? If food is hard to come by and you need to use all of your energy to catch or to find your food, do you think it would be wise to first run a couple miles around the block just to "exercise"? Or would you rather wait for that opportunity to inevitably arise when you'd *have to* run to catch your dinner?

Nowadays, places like Amazon and DoorDash do all of the running around for us, delivering everything we could possibly ever need right to our doorsteps. We have an abundance of food as well as many other conveniences all around. It's no wonder then that we no longer really *see the point* in moving when all of life's essentials are already taken care of. So naturally and unsurprisingly, our primal inner selves are just sitting around and waiting for that right opportunity to come along to inspire us to move our bodies, but the problem is, the right opportunity rarely comes along nowadays!

For a similar reason, it's also hard to *stick with exercise* long term. You will only sustain what you find pleasure in and *find purpose in*. If you don't enjoy something, or find gratification and fulfillment in something, then you simply won't keep doing it. And if you weren't even clear on *why* you started doing something in the first place, then the behavior really won't last. Eventually, you will realize that, as with getting started, you also don't see the point in *continuing*. Without a clear *purpose* for moving, you run the risk of defaulting back to your energy-conserving, resourceful yet prudent natural ways.

So does this mean that all is hopeless? Are we stuck in a perpetual mismatch between our basic human nature and our modern world? Are we destined to a life of Netflix binges and sloth-like lounge fests? The answer is a

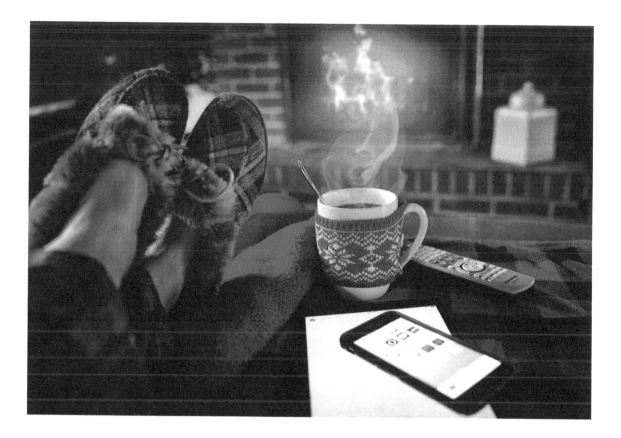

resounding NO! Our bodies were designed to move and to move often. Just because the reasons aren't always clear and directly right in front of us (e.g., being chased by a lion or our dinner running away from us) doesn't mean that we don't experience immense benefits when we do move our bodies. Not seeing any reasons in front of us does not mean there is simply no reason to move anymore.

Think of all the people that you've come across who have been able to build exercise into their daily lives. All of them have, at some point, made a conscientious decision to start exercising. They decided that exercise *did indeed* serve a useful purpose in their lives. And you can too. In fact, by reading this book, a part of you must already know there is an important reason to get moving!

The natural tendency to want to conserve energy for only purposeful movement is an *asset*…in the right environment. So as we continue, let us now get rid of the guilt. You, my friend, are not at all lazy, and there is nothing wrong with you. You have just been blessed with your ancestors' genes to carefully consider the need to move your body. Let us now do just that. Let us consider the critical need to move our bodies in today's world. Today's lion chasing us is not a lion in the literal sense. Today's lion comes at us in the form of a host of maladies and physical deformities if we don't get moving. It is *just as critical* to escape this modern-day lion, as it was to escape the real lions of our past.

Consequences of Living a Sedentary Lifestyle

Though we may not *want* to move unless and until we see the point in doing so, this does not mean that we *shouldn't* move. These days, the purpose of daily movement is not as obvious. It's a bit more abstract. No one is chasing you around (hopefully!), and your days of chasing the ice-cream truck down the street are probably long gone. But we *can* still make the reasons to move more obvious. As humans, we have the unique ability to act with foresight. We can *consciously* place these reasons in the forefront of our minds.

A sedentary lifestyle can increase the risk of:

> ➤ Cardiovascular disease and heart attack
> ➤ Stroke
> ➤ Type 2 diabetes
> ➤ High blood pressure
> ➤ High cholesterol
> ➤ Osteoporosis[1]
> ➤ Loss of muscle mass[2]
> ➤ Decreased cognitive functioning
> ➤ Certain cancers (colon, breast, uterine)
> ➤ Obesity
> ➤ Increased feelings of depression and anxiety

Do these consequences of being inactive scare you at all? I know that for many people, these diseases appear as just words on paper. But as a nurse, I can tell you that the way these diseases manifest in real life is very disturbing and highly unpleasant for all involved. These diseases can slowly creep up on you until suddenly, life, as you know it, gets turned upside down. No amount of pills can fix these cumulative issues once they hit like an avalanche. *This* is what makes them so scary and dangerous.

Benefits of Getting Moving

As with anything in life, dedicated practice is difficult to maintain if you are always asking yourself, "What's the point?" Well, the point is that there are tons of benefits that come with regular exercise. Let's take some time to review some of them, to remind you of what you will gain from this.

---

[1] Did you know that we reach our peak bone density at age thirty? Every year after that, it becomes a matter of using it or losing it. This is why it is critical to build up your reserves! The more stores you have, the longer it'll take for you to get osteoporosis or to experience bone loss. One way to help build healthy bones is with weight-bearing and strength-training activities.

[2] A similar story happens with our muscle mass. After age thirty, we lose 2–5% of muscle loss per decade! While we cannot totally prevent the natural progression of the aging process, we can control, to some extent, the *rate* of the progression.

One of the most common excuses people give for not exercising regularly (besides time restraints) is not having enough *energy* to exercise. But the paradox of exercise is that though it *requires* energy to carry out, it also *gives* you energy. Regular exercise can help you manage your stress better, make you feel more energetic, and help you sleep better.

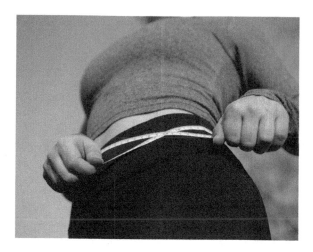

Additionally, not everyone who exercises does so for weight loss or to get stronger. Interestingly enough, one of the most pronounced effects of exercise is mood regulation. When you exercise, chemicals called endorphins are released. These "feel-good" chemicals give you an overall sense of calm, a feeling that is not all that different than painkillers. The catch is, you might have to wait until *after* the exercise is over to really feel these effects. And who couldn't use a dose of calm these days, right?

Exercise has the power to benefit your entire body. Other benefits of exercise include:

- ➤ Helps with weight loss
- ➤ Boosts metabolism and improves digestion
- ➤ Decreases insulin resistance
- ➤ Improves muscle strength and tone
- ➤ Decreases stiffness and pain from arthritis
- ➤ Improves heart health and reduces blood pressure
- ➤ Strengthens bones and decreases the risk of osteoporosis
- ➤ Improves cognitive functioning (brain health) by boosting mental clarity, focus, and concentration[3]
- ➤ Lifts mood with "feel-good" hormones, which can help with depression
- ➤ Increases overall energy levels
- ➤ Enhances sleep quality
- ➤ Decreases stress and anxiety levels

---

[3] As is the case with our bones and our muscles, we can also build up what is called our *cognitive reserve*. Think of the vessels in your brain as hoses. Exercise can boost circulation to the brain, clearing out those hoses of their cobwebs. Exercise can, therefore, improve cognitive functioning. Build up your cognitive reserve today to ward off some of the effects of the natural aging process.

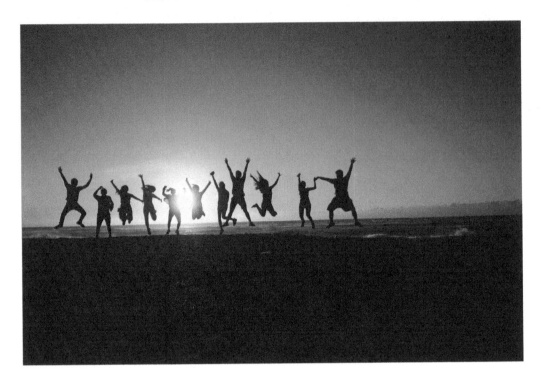

- ➤ Improves digestion
- ➤ Improves immune system functioning
- ➤ Increases joint, tendon, and ligament flexibility
- ➤ Increases self-confidence and mood regulation
- ➤ Improves posture, coordination, flexibility, and balance
- ➤ Stimulates the release of serotonin, dopamine, and norepinephrine (more feel-good chemicals!).

Feeling sluggish, low energy, grumpy, or anxious? Well then, it's time to get moving!

Exercise is a protective force against many unwanted chronic diseases. As we can see, the benefits of engaging in regular exercise are numerous. And don't think that just because you are X years old that it is too late to reap these benefits. My grandfather decided to join a gym for the first time in his life when he was eighty years old, and he loved every minute of it! Whatever your starting point is today, you *can* continue to grow stronger and feel better *no matter your age.*

Finding Purpose in Movement

In addition to knowing the many benefits of exercise and the consequences of being sedentary, it is also important to build some sort of *immediate* purpose into your everyday movements. For example, I try to always have a clear destination in mind when I go for a walk. When I play tennis, I see the point in moving my body because I want to win the game. When I do household chores (this counts as exercise too!), it is so I can relax in a cozy space later on. When I dance, it's for the sole purpose of having fun and letting loose. When I lift weights, I do it because I feel a sense of calm immediately afterward when my muscles relax. When I took up jogging, I did so because I wanted to keep up with my friends at a 5K we signed up for to benefit an animal sanctuary. A friend of mine kickboxes to release any pent-up frustration she may have and to deal with life's many stressors.

What can be the purpose of *your* movement?

How Much Should We Move?

As we begin to review the current exercise recommendations, please bear in mind that for now, you are focused on just building exercise into your life. A habit is formed not by *how long* you've been doing something but by *how many times* you've done it. And you're focused on finding something that you'll enjoy doing. Therefore, it's okay if you only do a few minutes per day in the beginning. The time and intensity levels can be increased gradually as your fitness levels improve.

This being said, current guidelines recommend strength-training activities are done at a moderate intensity *two or more days per week* and should involve all major muscle groups. In addition to muscle strengthening, it is recommended that adults sixty-five and older also incorporate regular balance and flexibility exercises at a minimum of several days per week to prevent the risk for falls.

Current guidelines also recommend that adults engage in 150–300 minutes of moderate-intensity aerobic activity OR 75–150 minutes of vigorous intensity aerobic activity per week.

Easy way to measure exercise intensity
A moderate intensity workout means that while you're exercising, you are exerting yourself enough that you can talk but not sing during a workout. This is called the "talk test," and it is used as an easy way to gauge the intensity of your workout. If your workout were *vigorous* intensity, then you'd barely be able to say more than a few words while working out.

Regardless of the duration or the intensity of your exercise as you are just starting out, remember that something is always better than nothing, and it is never too late to start!

*Quick Note on Reps and Sets

A repetition, or a "rep" is one complete motion of an exercise. A "set" is a consecutive number of reps. Completing one push-up means you've completed one rep. If you do 10 push-ups and then take a break, you've just completed one set of 10 push-ups.

How Should We Move?

Keeping things simple
PPL SHRG

Given the numerous options, it is common to feel confused or overwhelmed when it comes to having to choose the best way to move your body. And "people shrug" when they are confused, right? But with simplicity, there will be no need to *shrug* anymore. If you want to ensure that your body is able to sufficiently perform the basic functions of everyday life, learning the seven basic functional moves is a great place to start! As luck would have it, these seven moves can be remembered with the simple acronym: PPL SHRG—people shrug!

➤ **Pull**: This is any exercise that involves pulling movements, e.g., pull-ups and lateral pull-downs.

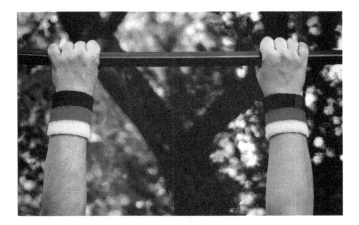

➤ **Push**: These are exercises that involve pushing movements, e.g., push-ups and dumbbell shoulder presses.

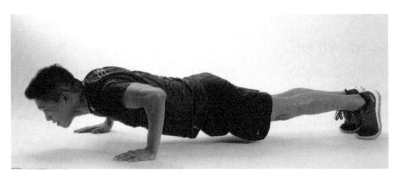

➢ **Lunge:** This is great for balance and stability, as it requires one leg to move forward (or sideways or back) at a time. As with squats, there's a variety of lunge exercises that you can try.

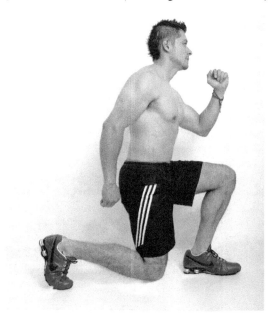

➢ **Squat**: Our ancestors spent a lot of time in the squatted position (natural floors can be dirty!). This is a great move to master, and there are many squat variations to keep things interesting. You can add resistance to the squat by incorporating weights.

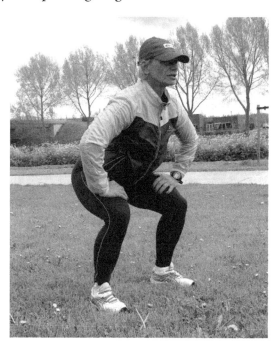

➢ **Hinge:** This is the movement you would execute when you bend over to pick something up (obviously an important one if you are clumsy!). Sample exercises are deadlifts and kettle bell swings.

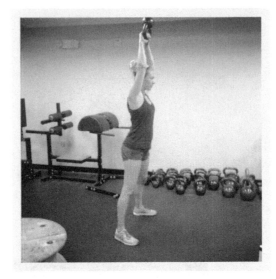

➢ **Rotation:** Life requires you to twist quite a bit. But not doing so properly can leave you injured. These are exercises that strengthen your core. Imagine a wood-chopping motion. That is an example of rotation.

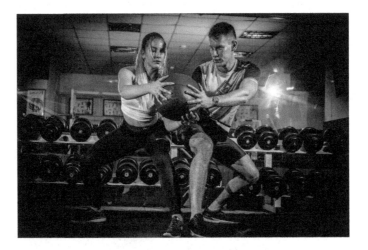

➢ **Gait:** This is the basic movement we call "walking." You think you are finished learning how to walk when you're a toddler. Think again! Many of us have poor postures from sitting and leaning over our screens all day. Stand tall and engage in this basic exercise as often as possible.

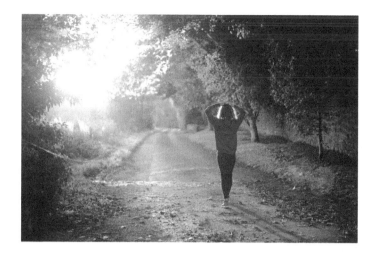

Make sure you are well versed on the proper form and technique of each exercise before beginning. Watch instructional videos, enlist the help of a knowledgeable buddy, or invest in a personal trainer. This step is well worth the investment and will pay back in dividends with your improved physique.

Any exercise that you do is essentially some variation of one of the seven key basic movements that the human body can perform. These are the basic building blocks of all exercises. Knowing this can go a long way toward simplifying your workout plan. You really don't need to be an expert on every single exercise out there. That is unrealistic and overwhelming. Just find some examples of exercises that incorporate these seven basic movements, and you are all well on your way to developing a fully functioning body!

Activity

✓ What scares you the most about staying sedentary?

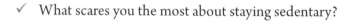

✓ Which benefits of exercise motivate you the most? Why?

✓ Do you feel fulfilled in life? If not, how can you create a sense of purpose or fulfillment, so that waking up each day becomes easier?

✓ What are some simple ways that you can add some *planned purposeful movement* to your daily life?

✓ To give you an idea of your fitness journey ahead, ask yourself how far off from the current guidelines are you. Spend a week tracking how much deliberate movement you partake in. How many minutes per day?

✓ How can you incorporate the seven basic functional moves into your everyday life? Can you sprinkle them into your day anywhere right now?

Part One Takeaway

You are right on track now, with the right mindset in place to proceed. We've established that it's not easy to move just for the sake of moving. We're naturally lazy, so our brains don't always like this. So don't rely on motivation or willpower to exercise, just to achieve an arbitrary goal a year from now. Instead, move with *purpose* and try to see the point in your daily movements. If you can add *purpose* to movement, then you'll rely far less on willpower to get moving.

Also ask yourself, as you age, do you want to *survive* or do you want to *thrive*? Disease does *not* have to be a normal part of the aging process. Increase your expectations of your own health. Reject negative stereotypes of aging. Disease is a combination of nonmodifiable risk factors *and* lifestyle choices. While *some* deterioration is a normal part of the aging process, we can, to some extent, control the *rate and degree* to which we age. One way is by exercising enough. In this section, we covered the consequences of being sedentary as well as the benefits of exercise. We discussed the importance of adding *purpose* to your movement. Are you sufficiently convinced yet to make this change? Make sure you truly are convinced before moving on to the next section.

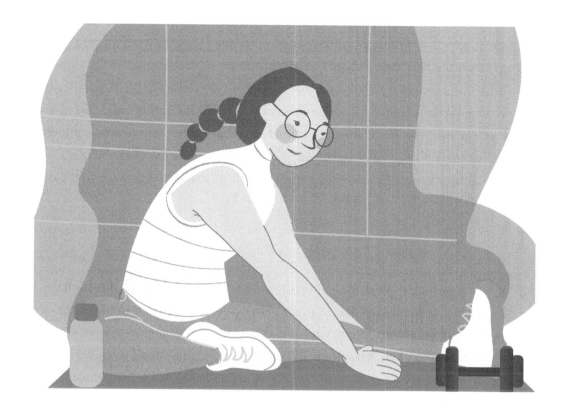

PART TWO

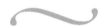

THE WARM-UP: BUILDING THE FOUNDATION FOR CHANGE

Hopefully by now, you are clear on the benefits of exercise as well as the consequences of being too sedentary. By having a better understanding as to why exercise can feel naturally unappealing, you also know that you can begin to work around this. You now see the importance of working *with* your nature rather than *against* it. You've learned about the most basic functional moves, and you see that this whole exercise thing doesn't have to be so complicated. You also know what you are aiming for, what the ideal amount of exercise is, according to current guidelines. Now we need to get into the weeds a bit, to ensure that whichever changes we make, they have a chance to last this time.

In order for any change to be successful, a foundation must be built. Think of this as the part where we prepare the soil bed for a new garden. You are creating an optimal environment for your new flower to flourish (a.k.a. your new habit). Checking on the garden and pulling the weeds (quitting the old habits) will be an ongoing process, as will be watering the new flower. But I promise it will get easier in time once your garden begins to blossom. So without further delay, let's begin!

STEP 1: EMBRACING THE NEW YOU

From this day on, you are going to take back control of your life by deciding which direction it is going to go. Gone are the days when you dread each doctor's visit because you didn't listen to his or her advice the last time about eating better and exercising more. Gone are the days that you have to passively and helplessly sit back and listen about how your blood pressure is still too high, your cholesterol levels are climbing, and the scale is tipping too far in the wrong direction, all because you didn't change anything since the last visit. This time, you'll beat them to it. You've already started to make meaningful changes!

Starting today, you are going to slowly start chipping away at becoming the best version of yourself. It is *never too late* to change. At any point in your life, you can decide to *identify* with who you wish to become. As was the case with my dad, one day he was a twenty-year-old nonexerciser, and the next day he became a *jogger*. Decide who you want to be and run with it!

But you must also accept that you will never be perfect. None of us will. It's not *happiness*, rather the pursuit of *growth* that will keep you showing up each day and living life to the fullest. And one of the best parts about this is that you are not only doing this for yourself…

When you take steps to improve your health, you are also doing it for those who care about you. You are doing it for everyone whose life you touch in some way. When you start exercising, you start to feel more alive. You will have more energy to actively engage with the world around you. The effects of exercise can also make you feel calmer and can leave you with more clarity. The ripple effect on other aspects of your life can be significant.

By decreasing one more risk factor of a lifestyle disease, you are also contributing to resolving a wider problem plaguing our society today. Lifestyle diseases account for a major loss of productivity and economic expenditure, not even to mention the loss of quality of life for so many. But by starting a healthy habits journey, you decided to say, "Not me."

Activity

✓ What exactly is it about the "old you" that you are looking to change?

✓ What will the "new you" be like? Look like? Feel like?

✓ Your identity and sense of fulfillment can come from many things besides your job. Practice changing your identity. This makes change all the more powerful. Who do you want to *be*? For example, you are not just someone who jogs. You *are a jogger.* You are not someone who just plays tennis. You *are a tennis player.* Or you can choose to be a yogi, a kickboxer, a weightlifter, or a walker. Who are *you*?

✓ Is there someone else in your life that would benefit from you getting fitter?

STEP 2: FINDING YOUR WHY

Any new change requires clarity as to exactly *why* you are making this change in the first place. Without clarity, there can't be confidence, and without either, there can't be motivation.

Are you doing this for yourself or for someone else? Being pressured by others to make a change is not always the best way to stick with something. Instead, see if you can figure out *your own* reason(s) for wanting this.

To help you uncover your reason for wanting to make this change, let's look at our most-common motivators in life. Almost every action we take is taken to fulfill one of our basic human needs. Our basic needs include the need for food, water, safety, security, stability, rest, acceptance, and intimacy. Deep down, it is quite possible that you are making this change to meet one or more of these underlying needs.

To uncover which basic human needs you're *really* trying to meet by making your new change, it's time to dig deep and do what I call, "The Toddler Exercise." I call this The Toddler Exercise because we all know that toddlers love to ask: "Why?"

You are not just exercising because you want to lose weight. What's the *real* reason? *This* reason will be your WHY.

The "why exercise" goes something like this:

"Why do you want to exercise?" Because I want to lose weight.

"Why do you want to lose weight?" So I can fit into that new dress.

"Why do you want to fit into that new dress?" So I can feel attractive.

"Why do you want to feel attractive?" So I can feel confident on that date.

"Why do you want to feel confident on that date?" So I can have a shot at true love.

So there you have it. What initially appeared as rather shallow motivation to just lose weight, turned into something far deeper—the need for love and connection. Let *this deeper reason be your motivation and your guiding light to sustain change.* Write this down!

Ex: "I am going to start exercising every day because I want to feel confident enough when I begin my journey toward finding true love."

Ex: "I am going to exercise more because I want to stay healthy and not get sick so I can be around longer for my grandchildren."

Ex: "I am going to build muscle so I can get stronger, and so I can continue to live on my own and not become dependent on others for my care when I'm older."

Activity

✓ What is the *real reason* you want to make this change to become more active? Use The Toddler Exercise to uncover your WHY, and write it out here.

✓ What does being healthy *mean* to you? Why is it important to you?

✓ What does being healthy *look* like? *Feel* like?

✓ Besides you, who else in your life will this new change impact or help? How?

✓ Find *clarity*: What do you want your future to look like? Where do you want to go? What do you want to do in life that this change will help you do? How do you want to feel? What's left on your bucket list? Surely you will need a healthy body to do these things!

Finding Your Pain Point

Part of discovering your WHY is discovering *what pains you*. What scares you? Sometimes we are more motivated in life by *avoiding pain* than we are in pursuing pleasure. There was a client who, for years, had struggled with becoming more active. At one point, she just stopped trying. It wasn't until years later, when she had her first grandchild, that she realized she couldn't bear illness or risk a premature death when her beloved little one was now in this world with her.

Your pain point might be dying young and leaving somebody important behind. Is the extra soda worth it? Maybe it's the fact that you might end up in diapers after a massive stroke, unable to communicate effectively with those around you? Have dementia and forget your loved ones and be perpetually trapped in your own mind? Not be able to travel anymore? Being on meds for the rest of your life? Dealing with the side effects... and the expenses? These are not meant to depress you, but they are also not far-fetched, unrealistic consequences. These are logical progressions of unhealthy lifestyle choices that I see happen to people all the time.

Activity

✓ What terrifies *you* about your current trajectory? Have you learned enough about what may be "down the road" if you don't make this change? Find *your* pain point.

✓ What are you willing to sacrifice today to make sure you don't experience this pain?

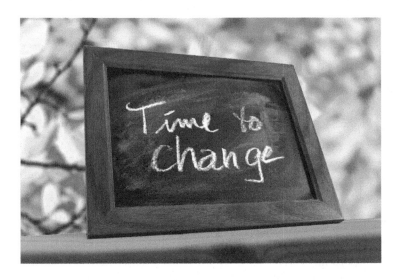

STEP 3: READINESS TO CHANGE...IS THE TIME RIGHT?

We all go through rather predictable stages when we make a change in our lives. We may not progress in the same order, and we may go back and forth between the stages. It is common for people to fluctuate *between* stages. Nevertheless, many people don't stick with change because they simply weren't *ready* to change to begin with. Their head wasn't in the game yet. This is why it is important to know *where you are* in the stages of change.

Mark a check next to the stage that best describes *where you are right now*.

Stage One: Precontemplation

You don't yet see the point in changing. You have no desire to make a change, and you think everything is fine as it is. You don't really see a problem with not exercising, and you feel okay for the most part.

If this is you and you've been told that you have unhealthy habits or your healthcare provider has advised you to make some changes, now would be the time to start understanding exactly *how* these habits might be impacting your life. Make sure you *truly* understand the consequences of living a sedentary life.

Tips to move on to the next stage:
What made you pick up this book in the first place? Let's start there. Do you see any *benefits* to making a change? Do you see anything in your current life that is not working for you or your health? Is there even a tiny improvement that you could consider making right now? Read about the risks of being sedentary and about lifestyle diseases. Consider the impact today's choices may have on you in the future. Then decide if a change is in store for you.

Stage Two: Contemplation

You are going back and forth. You know there might be a problem and a need for change, but you aren't totally convinced yet. You are still weighing the pros and cons of change. You are still thinking if change would be worth doing and if you can overcome the obstacles you might face when making a change.

Tips to move on to the next stage:
Make a pros and cons list of making this change. Also remember that the process we go through together in this book will make change slow and easy. You won't have to sacrifice all that you love in order to make this work. Work through your ambivalence to tip the scale in the direction of change.

Stage Three: Preparation

You've decided change *is* worth it, and your head is in the game now! You know you have to change, and you know that you are capable of change. Now it's time to start planning and even taking your first steps. You are planning ahead for possible challenges, and you are willing to tweak things with trial and error as you get started.

Tips to move on to the next stage:
Plan for action. Write out your goals, both short term and long term (we will do this together). Plan your very first baby steps. Think of what the bigger picture will look like, but to start, think about what small, easy things you can do to get started *today*. Maybe it's just planning a short workout. The idea is to start small and keep building from there.

Stage Four: Action

An object in motion stays in motion, and you're really making progress toward your goals now. You've got this! You've started making changes, and your motivation is strong. You're fully committed, and you're using your support system and your coping skills to push forward.

Tips to move on to the next stage:
To make it to the six-month mark, you will have to get good at foreseeing challenges and obstacles, which might push you off track from your healthy exercise patterns. Identify them and then plan around them. Keep your motivation strong by leaning on your support system, by checking in with yourself daily, and by revisiting your "why" as often as needed. And plan, plan, plan!

Stage Five: Maintenance

By this point, you've already overcome some hurdles. You've been working toward your goals for six months now, and you still remain focused and committed to your goals. But you also know that you can't totally let your guard down at this point either. Old habits can return with a vengeance. You still need to remember your "why," and you still need to check in with yourself and your progress often.

You can revisit this section as often as you need to during your journey.

Eliciting Change Talk from Yourself
When considering making a change, it is helpful to elicit what we call "change talk" from yourself, to continue on your path of convincing yourself that it *really is* time to make this change. One way of doing this is by creating a sense of urgency. Why must this change happen *today*? Why not tomorrow? Remind yourself that if you don't take action soon, your future will look no different than your present (at best). Would you be okay with this? You want a *life*, not merely an *existence*, to *thrive* and not just *survive*. The clock is ticking. Life is short. So ask yourself, why *now*?

Activity

✓ How would you like things to be different a year from now?

✓ Why are you deciding *now* is the time to change? Why not later?

✓ Think back to a time when you were more active. What was better about that time? How did you feel back then?

✓ What are the *best* things that can happen if you *do* become more active *now*?

✓ What's been stopping you from making this change? What are some of the obstacles you see ahead with becoming more active?

✓ How and why do you think this time you can overcome these obstacles?

✓ It's normal to be afraid or anxious to try something new. What are you afraid of? Name one fear that you have successfully overcome in the past.

✓ Were you physically active in the past? What did you used to enjoy doing? Was there something you were good at? Is there any physical activity you would be *excited* to start doing?

✓ Imagine your future successful (fit!) self showing up on your doorstep right now. What advice do you think he/she would give you?

STEP 4: YOUR EXERCISE HABITS AND ROUTINES

"Watch your thoughts; they become words. Watch your words; they become actions. Watch your actions; they become habits. Watch your habits; they become character. Watch your character; it becomes your destiny."
—*Lao Tzu*

You've probably heard it before, but it's worth repeating again: Humans are creatures of habit and routine. This is not a bad thing. Habits make us efficient. Habits allow our brains the opportunity to not have to think so hard about the tasks that we carry out each and every day. Habits allow us to go on autopilot so we can have leftover energy to focus on all the new stimuli around us each day. A habit can be brushing our teeth, having our morning coffee, walking the dog, or binge-watching TV every evening. Routines, on the other hand, are similar to habits but require a bit more of a concerted effort to carry out.

Why the focus on habits? Because it is habits and routines that shape our lives. They are what give our days structure. It's these little actions that we do each day that have the biggest impacts on our lives. And for this reason, each and every little thing you do really does matter!

Now, if you want to be healthy, you might label some of these habits as "good" and some as "bad." But keep in mind that there is really no such thing as a "good" or a "bad" habit. Habits don't have morals attached to them, so please don't feel guilty about your habits. Granted, a habit may be incredibly unhealthy or harmful to you but a habit in itself does not necessarily make you a bad person. So let's think of it this way instead; a habit is either moving you *closer* toward your goals or *further away* from them. *All* habits serve some purpose. If they didn't, then we wouldn't be doing them. So instead of asking if your habit is good or bad, ask yourself if a particular habit is getting you closer to who you want to be and where you want to go in your life.

How Exactly Does a Habit Work?

A habit is essentially a well-beaten path in our brains. The more you trod on that path (do the habit), the more reinforced it gets. At any time, it is well within your power to either continue down the well-trodden path or to forge a new path and let the old one grow over.

You spend your days either moving *toward* something you want or *away* from something you don't want. When the desire strikes to do either, you are *triggered* to perform an action, or a behavior. This is the *trigger* for your habit. This leads you to take action (the habit), and then you feel better because you've successfully moved toward what you wanted or away from what you didn't. In one way or another, you are *rewarded* for the action you took. And so you keep doing this action. This action is a cycle, and it becomes a *habit*.

Take, for example, my morning walk. For years, I have gone for a walk immediately after the last sip of my morning espresso. Finishing my espresso signals to me that it's time to get my shoes on and head out the door. I get restless if I don't (I *crave* the walk). So I go out and walk (the *habit*). While I walk, I feel less restless, I feel more relaxed, and I can feel my brain slowly waking up to the world around me. This is my *reward*. The health benefits from this daily walk are, of course, also rewards, but it's the *immediate benefit* of how I *feel* that keeps me going.

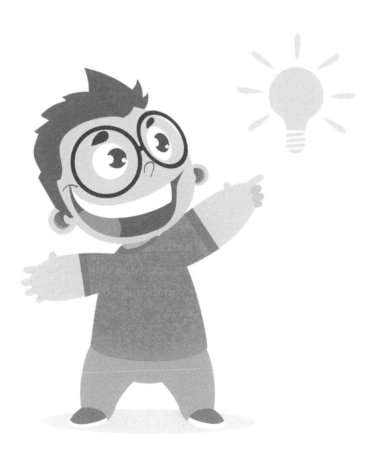

Common Exercise Cues/Triggers

The key to starting or quitting any habit lies in identifying the cues and triggers that *precede* the habit. Learn how to control or better manage cues and triggers and you are well on your way to adopting healthier habits. This is where the secret of habits lies.

Common exercise cues:

➢ Seeing your workout gear (or better, wearing the gear!)

➢ A reminder on your phone

➢ An accountability partner

➢ An activity that typically happens right before you exercise (e.g., my espresso)

Your Habits

Despite *knowing* all the benefits of adopting healthy habits and quitting unhealthy habits, why does it still feel so hard to change our habits? It's because by their very nature, habits keep us in our comfort zones. And comfort zones make us feel *safe*. I mean, who doesn't want to feel safe, secure, and have predictability in their daily lives? We all do.

So whatever the change, the trick is to do it in a way that feels safe and unintimidating, using small and easy steps to get started. And it means taking the time to form a new habit properly, with all its necessary components (trigger, action, reward).

You are going to focus on making only *one* new change at a time, *one* new habit to start with (in this case, a habit of daily exercise). No more setting unrealistic, grandiose goals that have you giving up before you even begin. No more biting off more than you can chew. That's just a recipe for failure, and right now we are aiming to succeed!

But first, it's time to take your habits off of autopilot and draw some attention to them. It's time to actively think about how you spend your time each day. Let's start with just your mornings. Write out your routine by making a list of what you do. Then, put a checkmark next to the must-do items (e.g., brush teeth, shower) and next to those items you deem "healthy." Put an X mark next to all other items. Then do the same for your evenings. You can use the questions below to help guide you through this activity:

Activity

✓ What are your current morning habits? Make a list.

✓   What are your current evening habits? Make a list.

✓   Do you have any midday downtime? Maybe just thirty minutes? Or a few scattered downtime periods? If so, how do you currently spend this time?

✓   Can you identify which habits are moving you *toward* better health?

✓   Which habits might be moving you further *away* from better health?

✓   After looking at your daily routine, when would be the *easiest* time to carve out time for exercise? If family obligations are an issue, can you include your family in your exercise time?

✓   Which current habit (that you will keep) can *trigger* you to start your new exercise habit? Maybe after your breakfast but before your shower? Maybe after work but before dinner?

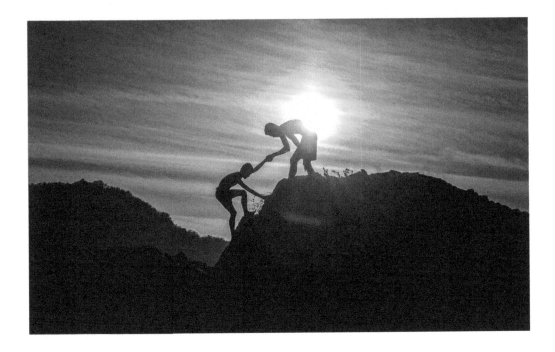

STEP 5: SETTING UP YOUR SUPPORT SYSTEM

Having a support system is highly beneficial when making any change. People who have support in place are far more likely to meet their goals. While it's not mandatory for success, it will definitely make things easier. Even better, see if someone wants to join this journey with you. There is also the option of working with a health coach or a personal trainer if you need that extra bit of support from a professional to get you going.

Basically, the idea is to find your tribe, the likeminded people who can support you and you them. And if you can't easily *find* your tribe, just create one!

Activity

✓ Name one to three people who can *really* support you in making this change. Make sure these are people you can count on to regularly check in with you on your progress.

✓ Is there someone in your life that you look up to or who inspires you, who's made similar changes to their exercise habits and succeeded? Who is this person? Can you reach out to them and ask for support/tips/advice?

✓ Think about how *specifically* your support person(s) can help you. Would a daily check-in work best? Would a weekly check-in be enough for you? Can you review the answers from this workbook with them? Can they exercise with you, maybe join you on your walks or meet you at the gym? Can they use an app with you so you can both see each other's progress each day?

✓ Which trackers/apps can you use to support and track your efforts, that can help keep you motivated in the beginning? This can include a FitBit, fitness apps, or even just an exercise log like what you will find in this book.

✓ Are there any Meetups, clubs, walking groups, or other ways to get active and meet more people at the same time?

✓ Is there a gym or a community college near you that offers classes?

✓ Is there an online community you can join?

Group workouts may or may not be your thing, depending on your personality. But these days, whether you are an introvert or an extrovert, there are plenty of options to choose from.

STEP 6: EMPOWERING YOURSELF TO MAKE A CHANGE

If you think you are going to fail at making this change because you tell yourself your willpower is low and you're just lazy, what do you think the chances are that you will succeed at making this change *this time*? I'd say slim to none. On the other hand, you are probably far more likely to stick with something when you believe that you have a decent chance at succeeding at it. This is why building confidence in yourself in the beginning can go such a long way. Don't skip this step!

Getting your mind ready for change can be half the battle when making a change. But even the slightest shift in perspective can work wonders. From this day on, you *can* change your inner dialogue. Tell yourself that you don't "*have to*" exercise. You "*get to*" exercise. You are celebrating all the amazing ways that your body can move. Exercise should never be used as a *punishment* for eating too much. You are *choosing* this, and you are empowering yourself to do something that you've been meaning to do. And you are *confident* that you can do this!

Activity

✓ On a scale of 1 to 10, how *confident* are you that you can make this change (10 being very confident)? Why didn't you choose a lower number?

✓ What successful changes in other aspects of your life have you made in the past? Which have you stuck with? How did you stick with them?

✓ Stories are powerful. Tell yourself a story to pump yourself up about what's to come. Convince your subconscious that you *can* make this change and become more active and that it isn't too late. *Tell yourself a short story of what the future you is doing.*

Example: "It's one year from now. I am on an airplane to go and visit my grandchild. I am able to stroll around the airport and not tire while I wait for my flight. I board the plane, and I effortlessly lift my own luggage over the overhead bins. For the first time in years, I don't need help. And best of all, this time when I see my grandchild again, I am able to bend over and scoop him up to give him a proper greeting, which he just loves. And then after all this, I still have enough energy to play with him for the rest of the afternoon."

Or...

"It's six months from now. I signed up for a 5K for a cause that I support, a charity that I believe in. A few of my friends decided to join me, and we have all been super excited for this day to come. A few months ago, I got short of breath just by climbing a few stairs. But little by little, I've been working toward becoming more fit. I started with walking, then jogging for brief spurts. Now I can jog almost the whole way. I can see the finish line ahead. Just a few more steps. I cross the finish line and am flooded with adrenaline, endorphins, and pride in this accomplishment. Today is a day I celebrate what my body can do."

Part Two Takeaway

Phew...in this section, you did a lot of very important work. Kudos to you for making it to this point! By now, you have embraced your new identity, you have uncovered the true reason(s) that you want to make this change, you've determined the stage of change you are now in, you've become more aware of your daily habits, you're prepared to mobilize your support system, and you have more confidence than when you started.

You have now built a solid foundation for change. This foundation is most likely what was missing in the past when you tried to make a change. This foundation will be your landing ground and a place you can return to if things get tough. In the next section, we are going to move just one step closer to taking a first action step. It's time to spring off from our foundation a bit and start really planning for our first steps. Are you ready?

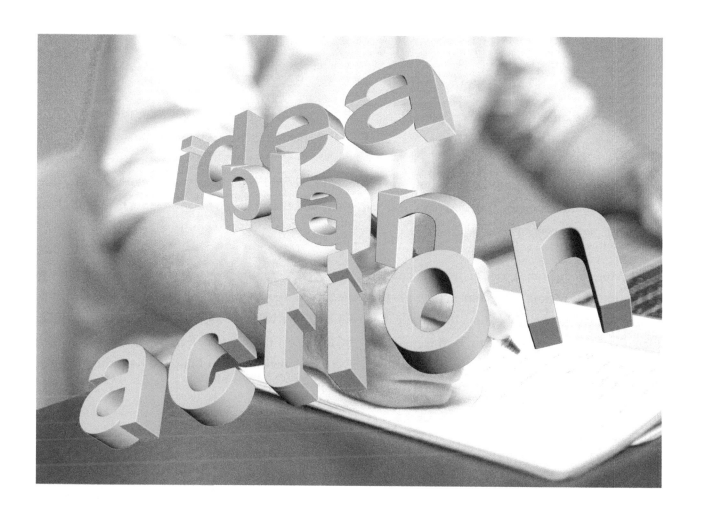

PART THREE

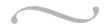

THE WORKOUT: GETTING
READY FOR ACTION!

Getting Unstuck: From *Planning* to *Action*

Undoubtedly one of the hardest parts of making a change is *just starting*. At some point, it's critical that you move from *planning* to *action* mode; otherwise, we can find ourselves stuck in planning mode forever. If you aren't mindful, planning can at one point just become an illusion of progress.

STEP 7: PLANNING AND TIME MANAGEMENT

I want you to ask one very important question here: Who or what are you most responsible for in this world? Who or what exactly do you prioritize, in terms of time and energy expenditure?

If you find that the answer to this question is everyone and everything under the sun, before yourself, then you simply cannot be giving your best to others. Something will eventually give if you are not *making* the time to care for *your own* needs every day.

Not having enough time is one of the most common excuses people give for not exercising on a regular basis. If you don't make fitness a *priority* in your life this time around too, then you will continue to get the same results. When we don't *make* time to plan our days, our lives lose balance, and life just happens *to* us rather than *for* us. Ask yourself honestly, by this point, can you truly say that your health and your fitness are now a priority in your life? If you honestly think it still is not, consider revisiting Part One, and return to this point when you are fully devoted to making time for fitness in your life.

Making Time

So in order to make this work, you must *make* time for it, not simply *try* to *find* the time for it. Exercise must be *prioritized*. You must see the value in exercising, and you must understand that taking this time for your health is not at all selfish. If you want to have energy to help others, and if you want to be a more vibrant being, then this is something that must be built into your schedule, every single day. If everything else under the sun comes before exercise and your fitness is seen as an afterthought, this simply won't work. Tell yourself that you *can* and *will* commit to this. Don't use the word "should" or say that you'll "try." Saying those words is just giving yourself an easy out. No easy outs this time. *You will do this because this matters to you. You got this*!

The Power of Daily Intentions

Going forward, you are going to begin each day by setting the right tone. After all, today is a fresh start, right? Our discipline and willpower are often highest early in the day. As the day progresses, we get *decision fatigue* after having to make too many decisions during the day. This is why making healthier decisions later in the day can be harder. For this reason, many people choose to make time for exercise in the mornings. It builds momentum, triggering the domino effect. If you had a smoothie and an amazing workout early in the morning, how likely is it you'll want to spoil the effects with fast food at lunchtime?

Setting aside time for yourself every morning to *mentally map out* your day is particularly important during the mindfulness stage of nurturing a new habit. And this planning time does not have to take much time. It is just a quick check-in. And as with any new habit you incorporate, it's important to make this process of a daily check-in with yourself very *easy*. To do this, you can use this workbook as your daily check-in. Just knowing that you opened it and completed an activity in it can confirm that you are on the right path each day.

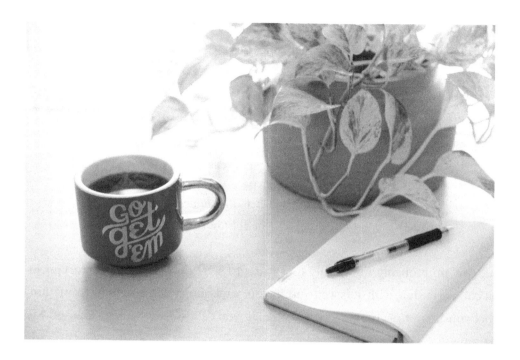

Your Daily Morning Practice

You are going to not just make a plan each day for yourself, but you are going to *imagine* carrying it out. This is called mental rehearsal, and it works!

First: Set a mental plan for the day. Ask yourself what you can *realistically* accomplish today, in line with your new health goal. By assessing your current habits and routine, carve out a new time slot to determine exactly *when* and *where* you'll take action toward your goal. If you must, remove a habit that doesn't currently serve you and use that time for your new exercise. Conduct your planning ideally at the quiet start of your day, before all the distractions and interruptions of the day set in. And don't be overly ambitious or you might just lose confidence and set yourself up for failure! If it helps, you can also write down your plan.

Second: Check in with yourself at predetermined times during the day to see how you're feeling, how it's going, and if you are still on track. You can set an alarm for this or just use a check-in time that cues you, like lunchtime. Use this time to remind yourself of your plan and *why* you are doing this.

Third: Review your day in the evenings: What worked? Where was your focus? Were there any challenges or setbacks today? What did you learn and/or what can you tweak to make tomorrow better or easier?

Keep in mind that making a healthy change is not just about making time to sit down one time to make lists, set goals, and name priorities (although this *will* be a part of your blueprint). Remember that nurturing a delicate flower requires *daily* attention and watering, and sometimes more than once per day. To build a new habit, managing your time *each day* and *mindfully checking in with yourself* has to be a nonnegotiable, ongoing process, each and every day, no matter what.

Pro tip: Our hungry ancestors woke up with the desire to get moving. Hunger hormones tell our bodies when it's time to go out and find food. Back in the day, food wouldn't come so easily, and it certainly wouldn't just land in our laps like it does today! So our hormones told us we were hungry, and those same hormones triggered us to get moving to find food. In today's world, you can still use this information to your advantage by planning to exercise when you're hungry. You just might find yourself more motivated to get moving!

STEP 8: SETTING REALISTIC GOALS

"True life is lived when tiny changes occur."
—*Leo Tolstoy*

By this point, you are probably sufficiently motivated to start exercising. It's important to make sure that whatever you choose to start with, it is well within your capabilities. If you choose something too difficult or something that you are not really able to enjoy, then it won't stick. Remember, slow and easy. You can grow from there, in time.

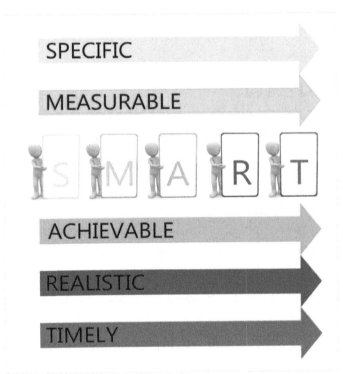

SMART Goals

When setting health goals, it's best to be as *specific* as possible. What *exactly* are you striving for? Saying you'd like to "become a runner" is fine and dandy, but we're lacking a plan here. To say that you would like to "lose fifty pounds" is also great, but it does not give you a clear road map showing you *how* to get there. Likewise, a goal of "working out more" is vague, doesn't let you measure progress, and it doesn't hold you accountable to a specific time frame.

This is why it's recommended to set what's called a **SMART** goal.
An effective goal is

Specific
Measurable
Achievable
Realistic
Time-bound

So basically, it has to be detailed. You have to be able to know if you are making progress. The goal has to be something you think you can actually do. It has to be aligned with your bigger, overall health goals. And you have to be able to accomplish the goal that you set within a realistic time frame.

Let's take running as an example: "I want to run a marathon by the end of the year." *How* exactly are you going to accomplish this? There are a million smaller steps that need to be taken in order to achieve this goal. This broad goal leaves more questions than answers, leaving a perfect opportunity for "analysis paralysis" and frustration to set in. If by the end of a couple months you still don't think you'd be able to run a marathon, there's a real chance you might lose confidence and begin to question your ability to ever achieve this goal.

So let's break this very lofty long-term goal into something more manageable. To convert this into a SMART goal, we could say: "I am going to run every Monday, Wednesday, and Friday morning before work for twenty minutes for the next four weeks." Then of course, you would gradually change this goal to include longer times and increased distances, in order to meet your ultimate goal of being ready for a marathon.

Once you've set your goal, it's time to make a promise to yourself to commit to it. Even if you don't manage to do the full thirty minutes in this example, consider any *attempt* at reaching thirty minutes a total win. *Consistency and gradual improvement are all we are aiming for when forming a new habit.* In time, the habit *will* be formed, and your performance *will* improve. Just be patient. One foot in front of the other.

Sample SMART Goals:
- "I am going to walk in the morning for ten minutes for five days a week for the next three months."
- "I am going to go the gym immediately after work on Tuesdays and Thursdays for at least forty-five minutes for the next thirty days."
- "I am going to do five push-ups every morning of the week for the next three weeks."
- "My goal is to run a 5K in under one hour by the end of August so I can improve my time from the last 5K."
- "I want to lose one pound per week for the next three months in order to lose about ten pounds before summertime so I can feel more confident in my new bathing suit."

Before setting your SMART goal, brainstorm a list of *enjoyable* exercises, a mix that includes strength-training workouts and cardio that you can really see yourself doing and enjoying. You can use the exercise index in the back of this book. The internet also offers an abundance of exercise ideas. A simple web search can really help get your creative juices flowing. Remember that a goal should be challenging but not too challenging. Remember to start with something doable. Start low and go slow as you create your goals. If your goal is too complex, grandiose, or unrealistic, you may lose confidence and may not stick with it. You can always return to this section and make new SMART goals as you grow. So are you ready to make your own first SMART goal?

Activity

✓ What is your SMART goal? Remember to make sure it's Specific, Measurable, Attainable, Realistic, and Time-Bound. Write it down here, but you can also make it more visible by writing it on a piece of paper and keeping it prominent in your living space.

✓ Set a date: This is your fresh start! Which day will you start your new exercise routine? Who can you announce it to, to make it more real? Don't forget your support system!

Adding your WHY to the end of your SMART goal can make it all the more powerful!

STEP 9: SETTING UP YOUR ENVIRONMENT FOR SUCCESS

Never overestimate how much self-control you have. Remember that at the end of the day we're all human. Most of us have much less willpower than we actually think we do. So when the time comes to do your workout, you want your living space to support your goals, not to tempt you to do something else.

Some people will choose to start their new exercise routine in a gym. What can be better than a space designed solely for exercise? But for others, for various reasons, going to the gym is just not feasible, or really all that desirable.

If your exercise will be taking place primarily at home, then it is crucial to invest time in setting up a space. A motivational space that is conducive to exercise is essential. Make this a space that you will *want* to spend time in.

Considerations

✓ Do you have a designated space to work out? Interruption free? Where can you carve out some space to do a variety of workouts?

✓ Are there any other distractions in this space that might tempt you to do something besides work out? Can you remove them? Make this a workout zone.

✓ What is the flooring like in your space? Will you need slip-free floor mats?

✓ Is there enough light and free-flowing air in this space?

✓ Can you envision different workouts happening in each space within your workout area? Our brains like delegating areas for different activities. Maybe one corner is for upper body strength training. Another corner can be for lower body exercises.

✓ How can you make this workout space your happy place? Is there anything inspirational that you can put in your workout space? Maybe exercise in front of a window? Or maybe you prefer a mirror? Perhaps your vision board? Your goals? Your intention statement? (Of course this workbook!)

✓ Is there a visible, high-traffic place where you can put your workout gear to make it incredibly easy to grab? Where is this place, and what can you put there?

✓ Can you play workout videos in this space? Play music?

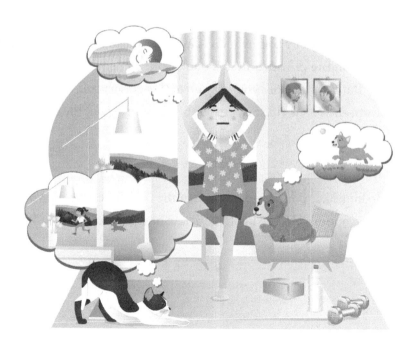

Tips:

Keep your workout space organized but efficient. A cluttered space is not welcoming. You can buy some inexpensive drawers and storage containers, and they can make a world of difference!

Mirrors can be beneficial in a workout area. Mirrors can, not only make the room feel brighter and larger, but can also help you ensure that your posture and alignment are correct, giving you live feedback.

To add inspiration, you can set up speakers to listen to upbeat stuff. You can have inspirational quotes up. You can hang nature pictures or beautiful artwork. Have fun making this space your own.

Your workout space doesn't need to be huge. There are plenty of exercises that don't require bulky equipment, for example, yoga, jump rope, or body-weight exercises like push-ups, sit-ups, jumping jacks, resistance bands, squats, or planks.

Don't forget that the great outdoors can also be your designated workout space! In this case, be sure to check out safe exercise tips for hot and cold weather. Remember, there's no such thing as bad weather, only bad clothing!

STEP 10: CREATING YOUR WORKOUT PLAN

Hopefully you are not filled with anxiety and dread when looking at your weekly workout plan. The idea again is to make this *realistic* and *doable*. Granted, in order to see and feel results, a workout will eventually need to be a bit challenging. This might take you outside of your comfort zone. But first we'll take it slow so we can just *form the habit*. This has to be something you know you can do, and rest days will be built in. Because this time we are *not* going to burnout or give up!

To begin, you might just want to start by adding more cardio into your week. Maybe later you'll add weight training, or vice versa. The template provided in this book is for someone who wants to begin with a well-rounded exercise program. But you can work your way up to this gradually if you prefer. Whatever works for *you*. For now, let's brainstorm answers to these questions before writing out the actual plan in your planner.

Activity

✓ What will your **cardio** look like? For example, consider the types of cardio activities, equipment needed, duration, pace/intensity; options include light, moderate or vigorous intensity. Write down some ideas.

✓ What will your **strength training** look like? Plan to do strength-training activities no more than two to three times per week, and space them out. You want to find exercises that target all the major muscle groups. Consider the types of activities, equipment needed, reps, weight (if applicable), and sets. Write down your ideas.

✓ What will your **flexibility/balance** activity look like?

Note: Decide ahead of time how many reps and sets you would like to do for your strength training workouts.

For general fitness, you can do 1-3 sets of 12-15 reps, with about a minute or a 1.5 minutes of break in between sets.

For muscular endurance, you can aim for 3-4 sets of 12-20+ reps with lighter weights. Keep breaks between sets short, at approximately 30 seconds to one minute.

To build muscular strength, do 3-5 sets using heavier weights but fewer reps, of 6-12 reps per set. Keep breaks a bit longer in between these sets, at approximately one minute or 1.5 minutes.

Structuring your week

Are you ready to try a healthy new kind of CARBS? The CARBS acronym is an easy way to remember how to structure your workout week with its necessary components.

C= **C**ardio
AR= **A**ctive **R**ecovery
B= **B**alance and flexibility
S=Strength training

First, you are going to choose one rest day for the week. No workout activities need to be planned for this day. Next you are going to choose two days that will be your "active recovery" days. Active recovery days are for gentle physical movements (e.g., yoga, swimming, long slow strolls, stretching/flexibility exercises, Tai Chi). Gentle movement on recovery days will help your muscles and joints rest and will prepare them to come back stronger for next time.

Now, choose the four days that you can realistically make time for exercise. Once you've chosen your four workout days, make a promise to yourself right now that no matter what, you will show up and put some effort in on those days. The absolute key is to start with slow simple steps to build confidence, build consistency, and form the habit! This point cannot be emphasized enough. Slow and steady wins the race! Just *build the habit.*

There are so many exercises and activities to choose from to help get you started. You can start with the seven functional moves. You can even start with just a few of the functional moves and work up to incorporating all seven into your routine. The idea is simply to get moving and to keep moving. Simple as that. Your body loves any sort of movement. And you don't have to block off a huge chunk of time to exercise either. Plan to scatter ten minutes throughout the day if that works better for you and your busy life. Just move. Any movement is better than none.

Use the Internet to help you brainstorm. Type in: "strength training sample workouts" or "cardio sample workouts." If you don't have equipment in your home and want to keep things simple, add "without equipment" or "using body weight" to your search.

Tip: You can combine cardio with strength training by doing circuit training.

Quick Tips to Get Moving
- ➤ Keep your gear ready to go. Make it easy to reach your gear, easy to throw on your gear, and easy to put away your gear.
- ➤ To get yourself started, commit to only two minutes of the activity to start with. If you feel like quitting after two minutes, it'll be okay. See if you can *just start*. And count *just starting* as success in the beginning.
- ➤ Whenever you have the thought to get moving, give yourself no longer than five seconds to get moving. Don't overthink it. For example, "I should get up and take a quick walk." Count down ... 5, 4, 3, 2, 1 ... tell yourself to just "go" and start moving. Don't overthink the urge.
- ➤ Remind yourself of how you will *feel after* the workout. You will never regret it.
- ➤ Don't wait to feel motivated. Move first. Motivation will follow.
- ➤ Turn off the negative self-talk. Leave no doubt in your mind. This workout *is* happening today.
- ➤ Remember what you already invested in this. You bought the gear. You've spent time on this book. You paid for that gym membership. You already told your friend you'd meet them for that workout. You've got skin in this game.
- ➤ Get rid of temptations to do other things. Turn off your devices. Don't use the Snooze button. Remove time-consuming apps (time-wasters) from your home screen.

A Quick Note About Normal Soreness vs. Pain

Normal soreness

It is critical that you be able to recognize the difference between *normal soreness* and *pain*. Normal soreness from exercise usually comes on twenty-four hours after a workout and should be gone after seventy-two hours. It is usually more generalized and does not feel sharp. It should not affect the way you move naturally, and the level of discomfort is usually tolerable.

Some muscle soreness is okay, and it just means that you did a solid workout. To minimize the *level* of soreness, try not to do too much too soon. Never skip the warm-up and cool down phases of your workout. Don't underestimate the importance of prepping your muscles for action, and then giving them time to transition back to a resting state. Doing so will go a long way towards preventing injury and soreness. Also be sure to vary your workouts to give your muscles time to recover. Do arms one day, legs the next. And on your recovery days, keep moving but perform lighter activities. This will help restore your muscles even quicker.

Pain

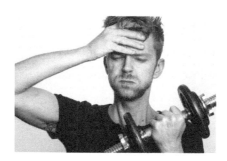

Forget about: "No pain, no gain." Invest in the time up front to learn proper form and techniques from a qualified exercise professional. Pain from exercise should never be overlooked. Pain from exercise usually strikes quicker than normal soreness and is more intense in nature. It may or may not occur during movement of a particular muscle. Pain requires attention and treatment, and you should never push through pain. Pushing through pain will only make it worse. Be sure to consult with your healthcare provider for any new onset pain.

Part Three Takeaway

Remember that on this journey you are going to be focusing on the *immediate* benefits of exercise. These are the ones you may not *see* right away but the ones you *feel*. Notice how quickly the human body adapts and gains strength. Appreciate your body for what it is capable of, regardless of the numbers on the scale. Be proud of your body when a workout begins to *feel* easier. Enjoy the feeling of your clothes fitting better, even though the numbers on the scale haven't budged enough for your liking. We are more than numbers on a scale. The human body truly is a gift.

While many people skip the foundation part of building a change, many others tend to *get stuck* in this last phase of planning and preparation. While this phase is critically important, there comes a time when you've planned enough and you are ready to start. We have now reached that time.

So congratulations! You finally made it! It is time for *action*. To stay on track, you can now start using the planner templates provided, until the habit of daily exercise becomes automated. To begin, you will find eight pages for weekly planning, to cover your first 60 days of forming a habit. This will give you a bit of extra support in the beginning. After the first eight weeks are over, you can start to use the monthly planners provided. You will have ten pages of monthly planning, to equal a total of one year, so your new exercise habits can be firmly set in place. While using your planners, you are welcome to simultaneously begin working on Part Four, to make sure the changes you are making really stick for the long haul.

Oh, and one more thing. Don't forget to consult with your physician before starting any new exercise program. Make sure you don't have any underlying medical conditions that could put you at risk. And after starting, if you experience any pain or unusual difficulty with any exercises, stop and consult your healthcare provider right away. Remember that each of our bodies is different, therefore no specific results can be guaranteed. While exercise offers a host of health benefits, it cannot replace medical treatment. With this said, use caution, learn proper techniques, start low and go slow and please don't forget to have fun!!

My Weekly Exercise Planner

My SMART Goal(s) with my WHY _____

_____

_____

☑ C= Cardio   ☑ AR= Active Recovery   ☑ B/F= Balance/Flexibility   ☑ S= Strength Training

Sunday	Monday	Tuesday	Wednesday	Thursday	Friday	Saturday
☐	☐	☐	☐	☐	☐	☐

My Cardio Exercises:

My Strength Training Exercises:

Upper Body: *Lower Body:*

My Flexibility & Balance Exercises:

After I exercised this week, this was how I felt:

	1= Poor	2= Fair	3=Average	4= Good	5= Excellent

Mood   1   2   3   4   5   Energy   1   2   3   4   5

Sleep   1   2   3   4   5   Wellbeing   1   2   3   4   5

What worked well this week?

What I would like to do differently next week:

My Weekly Exercise Planner

My SMART Goal(s) with my WHY _____

_____

_____

☑ C= Cardio   ☑ AR= Active Recovery   ☑ B/F= Balance/Flexibility   ☑ S= Strength Training

Sunday	Monday	Tuesday	Wednesday	Thursday	Friday	Saturday
☐	☐	☐	☐	☐	☐	☐

My Cardio Exercises:

My Strength Training Exercises:

Upper Body: **_Lower Body:_**

My Flexibility & Balance Exercises:

After I exercised this week, this was how I felt:

	1= Poor	2= Fair	3=Average	4= Good	5= Excellent

Mood   1   2   3   4   5   Energy   1   2   3   4   5

Sleep 1   2   3   4   5   Wellbeing   1   2   3   4   5

What worked well this week?

What I would like to do differently next week:

My Weekly Exercise Planner

My SMART Goal(s) with my WHY _____

_____

_____

☑ C= Cardio   ☑ AR= Active Recovery   ☑ B/F= Balance/Flexibility   ☑ S= Strength Training

Sunday	Monday	Tuesday	Wednesday	Thursday	Friday	Saturday
☐	☐	☐	☐	☐	☐	☐

My Cardio Exercises:

My Strength Training Exercises:

    Upper Body: *Lower Body:*

My Flexibility & Balance Exercises:

After I exercised this week, this was how I felt:

         1= Poor   2= Fair   3=Average   4= Good   5= Excellent

Mood   1   2   3   4   5   Energy   1   2   3   4   5

Sleep   1   2   3   4   5   Wellbeing   1   2   3   4   5

What worked well this week?

What I would like to do differently next week:

My Weekly Exercise Planner

My SMART Goal(s) with my WHY _____

_____

_____

☑ C= Cardio   ☑ AR= Active Recovery   ☑ B/F= Balance/Flexibility   ☑ S= Strength Training

Sunday	Monday	Tuesday	Wednesday	Thursday	Friday	Saturday
☐	☐	☐	☐	☐	☐	☐

My Cardio Exercises:

My Strength Training Exercises:

Upper Body: _Lower Body:_

My Flexibility & Balance Exercises:

After I exercised this week, this was how I felt:

| | 1= Poor | 2= Fair | 3=Average | 4= Good | 5= Excellent |

| Mood | 1 | 2 | 3 | 4 | 5 | | Energy | 1 | 2 | 3 | 4 | 5 |

| Sleep | 1 | 2 | 3 | 4 | 5 | | Wellbeing | 1 | 2 | 3 | 4 | 5 |

What worked well this week?

What I would like to do differently next week:

My Weekly Exercise Planner

My SMART Goal(s) with my WHY _____

_____

_____

☑ **C= Cardio**   ☑ **AR= Active Recovery**   ☑ **B/F= Balance/Flexibility**   ☑ **S= Strength Training**

Sunday	Monday	Tuesday	Wednesday	Thursday	Friday	Saturday
☐	☐	☐	☐	☐	☐	☐

My Cardio Exercises:

My Strength Training Exercises:

Upper Body: _Lower Body:_

My Flexibility & Balance Exercises:

After I exercised this week, this was how I felt:

	1= Poor	2= Fair	3=Average	4= Good	5= Excellent

Mood	1	2	3	4	5	Energy	1	2	3	4	5
Sleep	1	2	3	4	5	Wellbeing	1	2	3	4	5

What worked well this week?

What I would like to do differently next week:

My Weekly Exercise Planner

My SMART Goal(s) with my WHY _____

_____

_____

☑ **C= Cardio**   ☑ **AR= Active Recovery**   ☑ **B/F= Balance/Flexibility**   ☑ **S= Strength Training**

Sunday	Monday	Tuesday	Wednesday	Thursday	Friday	Saturday
☐	☐	☐	☐	☐	☐	☐

My Cardio Exercises:

My Strength Training Exercises:

   Upper Body: *Lower Body:*

My Flexibility & Balance Exercises:

After I exercised this week, this was how I felt:

	1= Poor	2= Fair	3=Average	4= Good	5= Excellent

Mood	1	2	3	4	5	Energy	1	2	3	4	5
Sleep	1	2	3	4	5	Wellbeing	1	2	3	4	5

What worked well this week?

What I would like to do differently next week:

My Weekly Exercise Planner

My SMART Goal(s) with my WHY _____

_____

_____

☑ **C= Cardio**   ☑ **AR= Active Recovery**   ☑ **B/F= Balance/Flexibility**   ☑ **S= Strength Training**

Sunday	Monday	Tuesday	Wednesday	Thursday	Friday	Saturday
☐	☐	☐	☐	☐	☐	☐

<u>My Cardio Exercises:</u>

<u>My Strength Training Exercises:</u>

    Upper Body: *Lower Body:*

<u>My Flexibility & Balance Exercises:</u>

<u>After I exercised this week, this was how I felt:</u>

          1= Poor   **2= Fair**   **3=Average**   **4= Good**   **5= Excellent**

Mood   1   2   3   4   5   **Energy**   1   2   3   4   5

Sleep   1   2   3   4   5   **Wellbeing**   1   2   3   4   5

<u>What worked well this week?</u>

<u>What I would like to do differently next week:</u>

My Weekly Exercise Planner

My SMART Goal(s) with my WHY _____

_____

_____

☑ **C= Cardio**   ☑ **AR= Active Recovery**   ☑ **B/F= Balance/Flexibility**   ☑ **S= Strength Training**

Sunday	Monday	Tuesday	Wednesday	Thursday	Friday	Saturday
☐	☐	☐	☐	☐	☐	☐

My Cardio Exercises:

My Strength Training Exercises:

    Upper Body: _Lower Body:_

My Flexibility & Balance Exercises:

After I exercised this week, this was how I felt:

	1= Poor	2= Fair	3=Average	4= Good	5= Excellent

| Mood | 1 | 2 | 3 | 4 | 5 | | Energy | 1 | 2 | 3 | 4 | 5 |

| Sleep | 1 | 2 | 3 | 4 | 5 | | Wellbeing | 1 | 2 | 3 | 4 | 5 |

What worked well this week?

What I would like to do differently next week:

My Monthly Exercise Planner

My SMART Goal

_____

_____

_____

☑ **C= Cardio** ☑ **AR= Active Recovery** ☑ **B/F= Balance & Flexibility** ☑ **S= Strength Training**

Month:

Sunday	Monday	Tuesday	Wednesday	Thursday	Friday	Saturday
☐	☐	☐	☐	☐	☐	☐
☐	☐	☐	☐	☐	☐	☐
☐	☐	☐	☐	☐	☐	☐
☐	☐	☐	☐	☐	☐	☐
☐	☐	☐	☐	☐	☐	☐

What is working well?

Are there any changes to make next month?

My Monthly Exercise Planner

My SMART Goal

_____

_____

_____

☑ **C= Cardio** ☑ **AR= Active Recovery** ☑ **B/F= Balance & Flexibility** ☑ **S= Strength Training**

Month:

Sunday	Monday	Tuesday	Wednesday	Thursday	Friday	Saturday
☐	☐	☐	☐	☐	☐	☐
☐	☐	☐	☐	☐	☐	☐
☐	☐	☐	☐	☐	☐	☐
☐	☐	☐	☐	☐	☐	☐
☐	☐	☐	☐	☐	☐	☐

What is working well?

Are there any changes to make next month?

My Monthly Exercise Planner

My SMART Goal

_____

_____

_____

☑ **C= Cardio**   ☑ **AR= Active Recovery**   ☑ **B/F= Balance & Flexibility**   ☑ **S= Strength Training**

Month:

Sunday	Monday	Tuesday	Wednesday	Thursday	Friday	Saturday
☐	☐	☐	☐	☐	☐	☐
☐	☐	☐	☐	☐	☐	☐
☐	☐	☐	☐	☐	☐	☐
☐	☐	☐	☐	☐	☐	☐
☐	☐	☐	☐	☐	☐	☐

What is working well?

Are there any changes to make next month?

My Monthly Exercise Planner

My SMART Goal

_____

_____

_____

☑ **C= Cardio**　☑ **AR= Active Recovery**　☑ **B/F= Balance & Flexibility**　☑ **S= Strength Training**

Month:

Sunday	Monday	Tuesday	Wednesday	Thursday	Friday	Saturday
☐	☐	☐	☐	☐	☐	☐
☐	☐	☐	☐	☐	☐	☐
☐	☐	☐	☐	☐	☐	☐
☐	☐	☐	☐	☐	☐	☐
☐	☐	☐	☐	☐	☐	☐

What is working well?

Are there any changes to make next month?

My Monthly Exercise Planner

My SMART Goal

_____

_____

_____

☑ **C= Cardio**   ☑ **AR= Active Recovery**   ☑ **B/F= Balance & Flexibility**   ☑ **S= Strength Training**

Month:

Sunday	Monday	Tuesday	Wednesday	Thursday	Friday	Saturday
☐	☐	☐	☐	☐	☐	☐
☐	☐	☐	☐	☐	☐	☐
☐	☐	☐	☐	☐	☐	☐
☐	☐	☐	☐	☐	☐	☐
☐	☐	☐	☐	☐	☐	☐

What is working well?

Are there any changes to make next month?

My Monthly Exercise Planner

My SMART Goal

_____

_____

_____

☑ **C= Cardio**   ☑ **AR= Active Recovery**   ☑ **B/F= Balance & Flexibility**   ☑ **S= Strength Training**

Month:

Sunday	Monday	Tuesday	Wednesday	Thursday	Friday	Saturday
☐	☐	☐	☐	☐	☐	☐
☐	☐	☐	☐	☐	☐	☐
☐	☐	☐	☐	☐	☐	☐
☐	☐	☐	☐	☐	☐	☐
☐	☐	☐	☐	☐	☐	☐

What is working well?

Are there any changes to make next month?

My Monthly Exercise Planner

My SMART Goal

_____

_____

_____

☑ **C= Cardio**   ☑ **AR= Active Recovery**   ☑ **B/F= Balance & Flexibility**   ☑ **S= Strength Training**

Month:

Sunday	Monday	Tuesday	Wednesday	Thursday	Friday	Saturday
☐	☐	☐	☐	☐	☐	☐
☐	☐	☐	☐	☐	☐	☐
☐	☐	☐	☐	☐	☐	☐
☐	☐	☐	☐	☐	☐	☐
☐	☐	☐	☐	☐	☐	☐

What is working well?

Are there any changes to make next month?

My Monthly Exercise Planner

My SMART Goal

_____

_____

_____

☑ **C= Cardio**   ☑ **AR= Active Recovery**   ☑ **B/F= Balance & Flexibility**   ☑ **S= Strength Training**

Month:

Sunday	Monday	Tuesday	Wednesday	Thursday	Friday	Saturday
☐	☐	☐	☐	☐	☐	☐
☐	☐	☐	☐	☐	☐	☐
☐	☐	☐	☐	☐	☐	☐
☐	☐	☐	☐	☐	☐	☐
☐	☐	☐	☐	☐	☐	☐

What is working well?

Are there any changes to make next month?

My Monthly Exercise Planner

My SMART Goal

_____

_____

_____

☑ **C= Cardio**   ☑ **AR= Active Recovery**   ☑ **B/F= Balance & Flexibility**   ☑ **S= Strength Training**

Month:

Sunday	Monday	Tuesday	Wednesday	Thursday	Friday	Saturday
☐	☐	☐	☐	☐	☐	☐
☐	☐	☐	☐	☐	☐	☐
☐	☐	☐	☐	☐	☐	☐
☐	☐	☐	☐	☐	☐	☐
☐	☐	☐	☐	☐	☐	☐

What is working well?

Are there any changes to make next month?

My Monthly Exercise Planner

My SMART Goal

_____

_____

_____

☑ **C= Cardio**   ☑ **AR= Active Recovery**   ☑ **B/F= Balance & Flexibility**   ☑ **S= Strength Training**

Month:

Sunday	Monday	Tuesday	Wednesday	Thursday	Friday	Saturday
☐	☐	☐	☐	☐	☐	☐
☐	☐	☐	☐	☐	☐	☐
☐	☐	☐	☐	☐	☐	☐
☐	☐	☐	☐	☐	☐	☐
☐	☐	☐	☐	☐	☐	☐

What is working well?

Are there any changes to make next month?

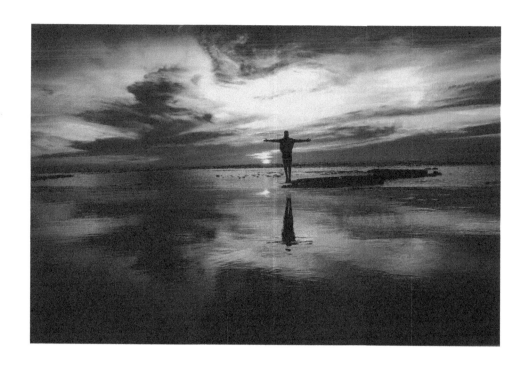

PART FOUR

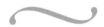

COOLDOWN:
SUSTAINING CHANGE

The Value of Perseverance and Discipline

Remember that habits lead to discipline, and discipline leads to success. In the beginning, motivation gets you going. In time, it is the habits and the routines that you build that will keep you going.

After a while of doing this whole exercise thing, hopefully less motivation will be needed to get moving. Exercise will feel as natural as the rest of your habits and routines. The ultimate goal is to be as disciplined with exercise as you are about brushing your teeth. The more you show up in the beginning with your tiny steps, the more the habit gets reinforced and the quicker it can be an automatic part of your everyday life. It's believed that it takes about two months for a habit to become automatic. Persevere through those first two months and you'll be well on your way.

It's also fine if exercise remains a *routine* rather than a *habit*. A routine simply requires a bit more intention and conscious effort to maintain, which this workbook has hopefully helped you with. A routine is something you make a point of doing each day. A habit, on the other hand, is more automated, and it will leave you feeling weird or off if it *isn't* done each day. So call it what you will, an exercise habit or exercise routine. The point is to keep at it and don't miss more than two days in a row.

But we all know that it is not always easy committing to a healthy change and sticking with it. It would be inaccurate to say that success *only* requires having strong motivation, a clear vision, and well-defined goals. There will be difficult days, and there will be challenges. There will be times when you question what you initially set out to do. There will be days when you question your progress and abilities. There will be days when you cave in to temptations and cravings. There will be days when you don't feel like exercising and you'd rather hit that happy hour with your friends. This is all expected. Life happens. It's how you handle and recover from the setbacks that determine whether you continue to succeed or whether you fall back into old behavioral patterns.

Foreseeing Obstacles

When the going gets tough, the tough get going. *Working through setbacks* is one of the best ways to *build your self-efficacy*. Reframe how you view a challenge, and see challenge as an opportunity for growth. A part of me changes every time I reluctantly complete a workout on days that I'd rather stay in my cozy warm bed. There's always that little voice inside my head that applauds me for pushing through. This makes me more disciplined. I feel stronger, and I have more confidence in myself, which then transfers over to other aspects of my life.

Foreseeing potential obstacles and planning ahead can help prepare you for when they inevitably arise. Predict which events might trigger you to skip a workout. Predict which feelings may arise that may challenge your desire to get moving. Predict what kind of weather may impede your workout. Predict the time restraints that may be imposed on you in the future. Perhaps you have work or family obligations. How will you work around these to *make* time for your health? Try to foresee these challenges and then brainstorm ways around them so they don't catch you by surprise. Life is always throwing curveballs at us. But the more you believe you're capable of working around them, the less thrown off you'll be by them.

Relapses can also happen even after a habit has been fully developed. It is all too easy to let the less-productive habits slip in, in place of the more challenging but healthier habits. Remember that missing several consecutive workout days can easily lead to complacency, and this can quickly become a slippery slope. Don't lose your momentum by not showing up. Keep that flame lit no matter how small the flicker gets.

All-or-Nothing Thinking

We often get caught up in this mentality that if you don't do something to perfection then it isn't worth doing at all. But a little bit of exercise is *always* better than being sedentary. Even small increases in physical movement can be beneficial. Be proud of any effort you put in. Don't fret over not completing the perfect workout, not working out long enough, or missing a workout here and there. *Don't be so hard on yourself.* If meeting goals were easy, they wouldn't come with such a great sense of accomplishment!

Fostering Patience

Growing a beautiful garden from scratch also requires patience. Don't rush the process. Rush the process, and you'll only end up frustrated. Behavior change doesn't happen overnight. It's a gradual process. The results of behavior change may not be *seen* right away. You will actually *feel* the results before *seeing* them. So just because you don't *see* results does *not* mean that nothing is happening. Manage your expectations and await the physical payoffs that come in time. If you are following your plan consistently and putting in an honest effort, then you *will* get results.

If you want to stay motivated for the long haul, focus more on the immediate benefits and less on achieving the end goal. With regard to achieving the end goal, just accept the notion of delayed gratification. When your focus remains on enjoying the ride, then there really is no rush to reach the destination anyway. Reward yourself along the way and find exercises that you truly enjoy.

The point of healthy change is not to stress you out, although *some* stress is beneficial because it promotes growth. *Too much* stress only leads to increased cortisol levels, which can be counterproductive for attaining optimal health. If your new changes are only adding stress to your life, perhaps it's time to realign your goals with your natural interests, strengths, skills, and abilities.

Dealing with Boredom

Let me ask you this: Is brushing your teeth *fun*? How about showering? Getting dressed? Preparing breakfast? Think of all the mundane things we do each day out of habit and necessity. They aren't necessarily fun, but we do them anyway because we see the value in doing them. Then why should exercise be any different?

It's kind of hard to make brushing your teeth any more fun than it currently is. But fortunately, unlike with some of our other daily habits, we can spice things up with our exercise regimens quite easily if we start feeling bored. It's okay to make adjustments as long as these adjustments are still aligned with our goals.

Admittedly, my workout routine does get boring sometimes. But usually, I find it's because I am not pushing myself enough. So I introduce something new. For example, I recently added wrist weights to my regular cardio routine. That added a whole new dimension to my workout. Then lifting dumbbells became dull, so I learned how to use resistance bands. Oftentimes, I'll go explore new trails, and sometimes I'll work out with a friend. I listen to new playlists, try new workout videos, and reward myself differently when I feel like I may be entering a rut.

Despite our best efforts to introduce novelty, boredom is still sometimes just a necessary evil. So I try to find ways *outside of exercise* to entertain myself in order to prevent *overall* boredom. Accept boredom as a fact of life and just let your mind wander during exercise, the same way you would when you are doing the dishes or taking a shower. You can use your exercise time to gather your thoughts or to unlock your imagination. In fact, my best thoughts and ideas actually come to me while I'm exercising.

Quick Tips for Success

- Accept the notion of delayed gratification.
- Accept that *some* sacrifice will be needed along the way.
- Foresee obstacles and plan ahead.
- Reflect on how far you've already come (improved health markers, weight loss, strength gains, endurance, feeling better, etc.).
- Build discipline by not allowing yourself to miss days.
- Build resilience by pushing through. This will make you stronger.
- Overcome setbacks and relapses quickly so momentum continues.
- Keep improving your performance.

Getting Back on Track

Let's say you let a few days go by where you didn't exercise at all. Maybe you were feeling under the weather. Or maybe life just happened. A few days turned into a few weeks, which quickly turned into a few months. How in the world do you get back on track after this?

First of all, forgive yourself for slipping off track. Accept it for what it is. It's okay. Everyone has slip-ups. You know you are soon going to be back at it, and today is a new day to begin again. There is no rule that says you can't keep trying an infinite number of times if you must!

Remember that this whole healthy living thing is a *journey*. For as long as you are alive, there is no end date. So we just move on. Try to learn *why* you slipped and plan on doing things a bit differently the next time. *Revisit this book.* Start from the beginning if you must. Pump yourself up all over again. Go through the motions. Rebuild your confidence. Find your support again, your tribe, if you will. Revisit your WHY. Write new goals, and prepare a fresh new soil bed for the next spring to come again. There is *always* another spring on the horizon. And as with all gardens, yours, too, will begin to flourish once again.

Activity

✓ What will you do if you start to dread your workouts?

✓ What if your workouts start feeling boring? How can you make your workouts more fun or more challenging?

✓ What is this exercising *today* going to get you in the *future*? Are you willing to wait for those results and sacrifice a bit today for that? When else have you delayed gratification?

✓ Have you ever been able to stick with something in the past, knowing you'd be rewarded later in the future?

✓ How will you get back on track if you skip a few workouts in a row? (The key is to try to *not* skip days!)

✓ What has stopped you in the past from sticking with exercise? How will this time be different?

✓ If you exercise outside, how will you keep up with your workouts during bad weather days?

✓ How will you notice that you've slipped off track?

✓ What is your plan if you totally slip off track? What will you do *first* to get back on track again?

You've Got This!

The ability to push through adversity is what helps build grit, perseverance, and resilience. *Develop coping skills* that can help get you closer to your goals. Engage in positive self-talk. Continue telling yourself that while pushing through may initially *feel* like you are making a sacrifice, you will *never* regret having engaged in a healthy activity at the end of the day.

You may find yourself pleasantly surprised that while you set out to achieve certain goals, other unexpected benefits may spring up. Check in with yourself often and do not focus on any one single outcome. As often as needed, reassess the alignment of your daily actions with your long-term goals. Squash that nonsense negative self-talk that questions your motives for healthy change. Instead, remind yourself of all of your unique strengths and abilities and of the bright future ahead of you as your body continues to get stronger. Easier said than done I know. But with practice comes success. Do not stray from your path. You *will* get there if you want something badly enough.

Hopefully on this journey, you've learned the importance of creating the right habits and systems to organize your life. Systems and processes aligned with SMART goals equal success! You've also learned that it's your daily habits and routines that bring you closer to your goals that make a life well lived.

Final Words

It is true that breaking a bad habit can feel a bit like pulling weeds in a garden. It may look easy at first, but then you discover that the roots are firmly planted and intertwined deep beneath the soil. But I also hope that you begin to see how building healthy habits can be as rewarding a process as growing your own beautiful garden. Eventually, by sheer strength and number, the plants and flowers that you nurture will overtake those pesky weeds, and in the end, you'll have yourself a beautiful, healthy garden to show for!

Now imagine what your life could eventually look like if you *don't* sustain this healthy change, if you let the figurative weeds take over the garden you spent so much time tending to. Inevitably, the consequences of living a sedentary life will catch up to us all. Without enough use, our bodies become weak and frail.

As you age, this could possibly manifest to mean medical copays, doctor's appointments, lifestyle diseases, low energy, aching joints, weak muscles, low endurance, reliance on assistive devices, dependence, inability to care for yourself physically, inability to help others, decreased productivity, and higher risk for falls, just to name a few! Is this okay with you? It doesn't have to be.

Instead, you can choose to age gracefully. You can maintain your independence, you can stay strong, and you can welcome each day being the vibrant person that you've chosen to be. You can live with intention and decide *this* is the life you want. You can decide that *you* will be one of the ones who age with *vigor*. A life lived with focus on what's important and with intention is a life well lived. You've taken control of your life because you want better for yourself. And at the end of the day, there is nothing more fulfilling than this.

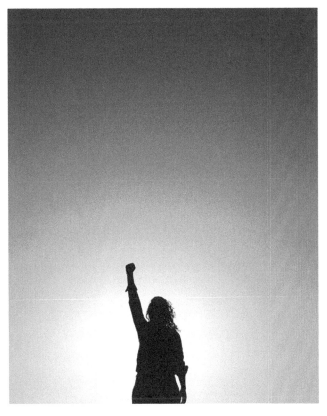

Accept that there will be days ahead when you will not feel like springing out of your bed in the mornings to do those Burpees. There will still be days when you are tempted to take that short-cut back home on your daily walk. There will be those instances when you will count on your natural lazy gene to get you through a day's activities. In those moments, remember that you are human. In fact, I want you to remember that it is *because* you are human and resourceful that those moments occur. Be proud and unapologetic about this. Embrace your laziness gene. And once you've accepted that this is a part of who you are, then I want you to turn that *thinking* and *planning* part of your brain back on again and remember why you started this journey in the first place. Remember that you are *also* now a fit person, a healthy person, and a regular exerciser.

If you've come this far, this means that you have designed a *system* for yourself. If you followed all of the steps, then this is a system that *works*. It overrides your lazy gene for a greater purpose. Your system is fueled by your WHY. Your system was customized, and it's a system that you know how to tweak accordingly to meet your needs and desires. You know what works and what doesn't. You know the power of daily habits and small steps. You know how to make a change when you need to. You've also gotten to know yourself a bit more on this journey, and with this knowledge, you feel empowered. Your entire outlook on active living has been redefined. You know how to hack that lazy gene and celebrate the gift of moving your body and all the benefits you can reap from this. Even better, you know how to make this happen, *consistently*.

Though critically important, exercise is only one piece of the healthy living puzzle. There are a whole host of benefits to moving your body more often. But there's more to it. *Fueling* your body with what it needs to perform well is equally important. And your diet also really matters when it comes to weight management. Healthy eating is another critical piece of the healthy living puzzle. If you think you would benefit from a little more help with adopting healthy eating habits, be sure to check out **AndiamoFit's *Healthy Eating Habits.***

My Weekly Exercise Planner

My SMART Goal(s) with my WHY _____

_____

_____

☑ C= Cardio   ☑ AR= Active Recovery   ☑ B/F= Balance/Flexibility   ☑ S= Strength Training

Sunday	Monday	Tuesday	Wednesday	Thursday	Friday	Saturday
☐	☐	☐	☐	☐	☐	☐

<u>My Cardio Exercises:</u>

<u>My Strength Training Exercises:</u>

    Upper Body: *Lower Body:*

<u>My Flexibility & Balance Exercises:</u>

<u>After I exercised this week, this was how I felt:</u>

	1= Poor	2= Fair	3=Average	4= Good	5= Excellent

Mood	1	2	3	4	5	Energy	1	2	3	4	5
Sleep	1	2	3	4	5	Wellbeing	1	2	3	4	5

<u>What worked well this week?</u>

<u>What I would like to do differently next week:</u>

My Monthly Exercise Planner

My SMART Goal

_____

_____

_____

☑ **C= Cardio**   ☑ **AR= Active Recovery**   ☑ **B/F= Balance & Flexibility**   ☑ **S= Strength Training**

Month:

Sunday	Monday	Tuesday	Wednesday	Thursday	Friday	Saturday
☐	☐	☐	☐	☐	☐	☐
☐	☐	☐	☐	☐	☐	☐
☐	☐	☐	☐	☐	☐	☐
☐	☐	☐	☐	☐	☐	☐
☐	☐	☐	☐	☐	☐	☐

What is working well?

Are there any changes to make next month?

BONUS EXTRAS

Quick tips on how to get unstuck: From *planning* to *action*

You can hang this up in a visible place in your home to keep you moving!

❖ Remember that the more clarity you have, the less confidence you'll need. Are you clear on your WHY?

❖ Stop waiting to feel motivated to take action. We've got it all backwards. It's the other way around. Your motivation will come from the actions you take. Move first and then you *will feel motivated* to continue. Start with one tiny step.

❖ Planning does not equal progress. Endless prepping is just an illusion of progress. It is time to get moving.

❖ Review your vision of your future self once more. Imagine your future self as often as you need to while on this journey!

❖ Regardless of how unmotivated you *feel*, plan to do something ridiculously easy toward your goal *every single day*. Accept that you won't *always* feel motivated … but promise yourself you'll show up anyway. It's about keeping momentum going. It's much harder to *restart* something when you've lost momentum.

❖ Stop trying to be a perfectionist. Get rid of that all-or-nothing thinking. A little bit of movement is always better than none. Accept that you might suck at something new. We all have to start somewhere. You'll get better in time. Keep at it.

❖ Remember the two-minute rule—commit to doing the activity for just two minutes, and tell yourself that something is better than nothing. Just show up. I can almost assure you that you will go longer than those two minutes just about every time.

❖ Track any and all progress, including (and especially!) *just showing up* for the workout.

❖ Don't skip days. Show up for every *planned* day, even if you have to give less effort. Don't break the habit.

❖ Remember that you won't have to rely on willpower as much once a habit becomes more automated. Eventually, your new habit won't be new anymore, and it will seem as easy as brushing your teeth! In fact, you will eventually feel off if you *don't* perform the new habit.

❖ Make it desirable to move. It's even easier to kick into action mode when you get to engage in an activity you enjoy.

❖ Rather than devote a chunk of time to exercise each day, you could also try "snacking on exercise." It's a mental trick. It's much easier to get moving when you know you have a smaller workout in front of you. You can try this by simply adding movement throughout your day, sprinkling in exercise every opportunity you get. I, for example, use my stepper in the mornings in between tasks. I use my resistance band on work calls. I do a set of squats before I refill my coffee. I go on walking meetings. Little chunks of purposeful movement add up during the day. Just be sure to track how much you've done.

❖ Even if you exercise regularly, once per day, there are still negative effects to spending too much time the rest of the day lounging around. There are plenty of apps and trackers that can remind you to get up and stretch or move every hour. But if you like to keep things simple, just set an alarm on your phone. Or use environmental cues/reminders.

❖ Think of how you will feel *after* the workout. And remember that you'll always regret not having shown up but will never regret having shown up.

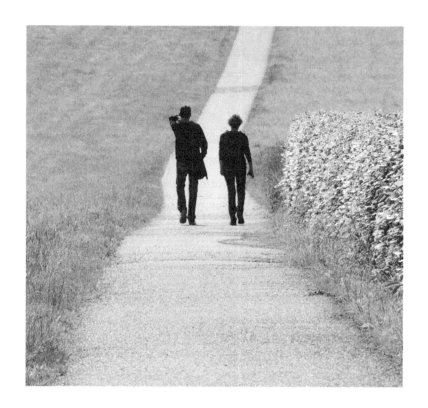

BASIC WALKING
PROGRAM GUIDE

How to begin a walking program

Quite simply, a regular walking routine is one of the best things you can do for your health. Fortunately, it's also one of the *easiest* activities to begin. You can apply all that you have learned so far about habits and getting started and apply it to a walking routine. Contrary to popular belief, walking *can* be a great cardio workout.

Here are the most common barriers people cite for not walking enough, along with ways to overcome them:

The weather sucks!

Weather doesn't suck, only your clothing does. Wear short sleeves on a crisp fall day, and you'll be cold. Don't blame the beautiful autumn weather. It's simply a clothing mismatch.

Fear

Fear of falling. Fear of strangers. Fear of ne'er-do-wells. Unfortunately in today's world, this one's a legitimate concern regardless of where you live. I personally can't let fear stop me from doing things I value and things I love; otherwise, I would never leave the house. I've traveled the world and walked alone through all sorts of neighborhoods (good and not so good), and somehow I'm still here (luck, perhaps?). Trust your gut. Be aware of your surroundings at all times. Inform loved ones where you're going. Bring someone (or a pet) along with you. Bring your phone. Carry a whistle or an alarm. The point is you can work around this one too by taking the right precautions. The reward is well worth the potentially small risk in my opinion.

You have no destination in mind and therefore don't see the point in walking.

As humans, we need to see the point in doing something before we do it. In theory, we know walking is good for us. But we need more than that. We need an immediate reward. Plan a destination and feel a sense of accomplishment when you arrive.

Walking is too slow. It's better to drive.

Sure, but then you won't get any of the benefits! Driving simply does not offer any of the health benefits that walking does!

You don't have enough nice walking paths nearby

Keep things simple. The idea is to move your body and get fresh air, safely, of course. Go and scope out a decent area. It doesn't even have to big because you could do a few loops. Where there's a will there's a way. If I can make pitiful loops around the parking lot of an old office complex during the day, I have faith that you can also find something that works for you. Heck, you can even see if your job can consider having walking meetings outside!

Chronic pain

This is a trickier one. This one will depend on what kind of pain you have and where it is. If it's knee pain, you might have to start low. You might need to visit an orthopedist to get inserts. You might even need medical intervention before you continue. But whatever it is, address it. The day you stop walking is the day your countdown begins toward immobility and dependence. And it happens fast.

It's boring

With today's technology, there are a million and one ways to spice things up. Listen to music with your favorite playlist. Listen to an interesting podcast. Call a friend. Or better yet, invite one along with you. Or simply clear your mind and then see where it wanders off to as your body does the same.

Ten easy tips on how to get started:

1. Be clear on the reason you're creating a walking routine. Keep your WHY at the forefront of your mind. Are you walking *away* from disease? Are you walking *toward* better health? Whatever it is, remind yourself of your underlying WHY on those cold, dark, rainy, hot, and otherwise bad weather days in order to keep yourself focused and driven.

2. Get hyped! Grab your gear and get it all set to go. The beauty of walking is that you really don't need much gear in order to get started.

3. Map out your route ahead of time. When you walk out your door, know exactly where you are headed and then head there with confidence. Sure, aimlessly wandering can be fun but a walk without a destination might be a bit intimidating when you are first starting out. Confidence will take you farther than you probably even planned to go!

4. When you're first starting out, plan to walk a shorter distance than you know you can do: start low and go slow; this too will boost your confidence for the next walk. You can do this by starting with just a five or ten-minute walk.

5. Remember that in the beginning, it's all about *just starting* the habit. In the beginning, your goal is not accomplished by measuring the distance or the speed of your walk (all that can come later when you're a pro). Right now, give yourself points just for heading out.

6. Gradually increase your pace and distance to what feels comfortable. A brisk pace is 3 or 3.5 mph. This is a mile in about seventeen to twenty minutes. If you want to incorporate more cardio, try your hand at power walking. You know you're getting a cardio workout when it becomes difficult to carry on a normal conversation.

7. Have fun! Talk to your neighbors (if that's your thing). Listen to music or podcasts. Or do what I do and just absorb the nature around you. Appreciate nature's beautiful melodies and practice gratitude for the smallest pieces of beauty all around.

8. Incorporate walking whenever and wherever you can throughout the day. It could even be during your lunch break. Then make note of how energized you feel when you return to your work!

9. Always be mindful of how you feel *before* and *after* you return from a walk. Note the positive effects it has on your mood, energy levels, perspective, mindset, etc. THIS is what will keep you coming back for more.

10. Don't strive for perfection. You *will* miss days (unless you're like me and your dog won't let you …). Just try not to miss two days in a row. Make the walk shorter if need be, but don't miss more than two days (barring illness or injury, of course).

As you begin your walking habit, remember that any bit of movement is better than none, and it's never too late to start. Any walk you take is a success. But as you progress, you will want to do a bit more, for added health benefits. You do this by gradually adding five minutes of walking time per week. Eventually, you will work your way up to a minimum of thirty minutes of walking, six days per week.

Your Walking Plan

I will start walking because_____
(What is your biggest motivator to start walking? Is it a health scare? To lose weight?)

➤ **When I will walk:**

➤ **My route and how far I will walk:**

➤ **Gear I need to prepare:**

➤ **How I can make walking fun and rewarding:**

➤ **How will I feel right after my walks?**

Quick Guide: Fifteen Ways to Be More Active at Work

- Set an alarm every hour to get up and walk around.

- Consider having walking meetings.

- See if your boss will invest in a standing desk for you.

- Count your steps (with an app or a simple pedometer).

- Use part of your lunch break to take a walk.

- Get a headset for phone conversations and walk while you talk.

- Don't send that email. Get up and walk over to your colleague's desk.

- Engage in simple, quick exercises, often. Carry a resistance band with you. Do some quick squats, jumping jacks, wall push-ups, or chair dips.

- Create reasons to move and create a work environment that makes you get up. Don't keep everything within easy reach at your desk.

- Make sure your clothes are comfortable (enough) to move around in.

- Create mini habits. Reward yourself with a little walking break after a difficult task. Reward yourself with a stretching break after an intense meeting. Get up at the top of every hour (or other cue).

- Intentionally choose destinations farther in mind. Use the bathroom farther down the hall. Take the steps. Park farther away.

- Consider getting a desk cycle or a treadmill desk.

- Switch out your old office chair for an exercise ball instead to engage your core.

- Use your commute time and the minutes before/after your commute to squeeze in more movement where you can. Stand in the train rather than sit.

- Get off the bus one stop sooner. Walk the halls of your office, or better yet make a quick loop around the building before getting to your desk. Plan for this little bit of extra time each day. It's worth it.

EXERCISE INDEX

Quick tips:

✓ Exhale during exertion.

✓ Use the two-minute rule to get started.

✓ Recognize the difference between soreness and pain.

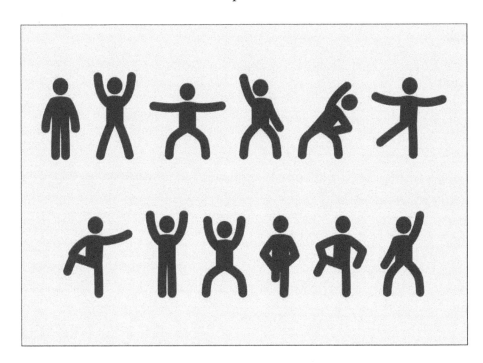

Included is a sample of the most common exercises. It is crucial to learn how to execute proper form and technique in order to prevent injury and to get maximal gains. There is no shortage of YouTube videos to demonstrate proper techniques, or you could hire a personal trainer to help get you started. Experiment with different exercises that you can do and that you enjoy. Be sure to include exercises that work your upper body, your lower body, and your core, as well as those that promote flexibility and balance. Keep in mind the current exercise guidelines when planning your exercise routine.

Stretching Exercises

➢ Shoulder blade squeeze

➢ Pelvic tilts

➢ Toe taps and heel raises

➢ Knee lifts

➢ Shoulder and upper-back stretch

➢ Ankle rotations

➢ Neck stretch

➢ Upper back/dive stretch

➢ Inner-thigh stretch

Balance and Flexibility Exercises

➢ Single-leg balance

➢ Tree pose

➢ Tightrope walk

➢ Flamingo stand

➢ Lunges

➢ Bicycle crunch

➢ Tai Chi

➢ Standing leg lifts

Chair Exercises

➢ Knee lifts

➢ Toe taps

➢ Heel raises

➢ Shoulder circles

➢ Hand stretches

➢ Tummy twists

➢ Side bends

➢ Leg extension

Cardio Exercises

➢ Jumping rope

➢ Jumping jacks

➢ Speed walking, jogging, running

➢ Swimming

➢ Steps/step-ups

➢ Cycling

Strength-Training Exercises (with equipment)

Using resistance bands or dumbbells:

Upper body exercises: Bicep curls, triceps extensions, wrist curls, upright front row, overhead shoulder press, chest fly, lateral raises and front raises, bent-over row, shoulder shrug, chest/bench press, lateral and front pull-down, Romanian deadlift, clean and press, lying dumbbell fly, kettlebell swings and transfers

Lower body with resistance bands: *On ground:* Leg press, fire hydrant, glute kickbacks, clamshell. *Standing:* resistance-band squats, leg lifts, glute kickbacks, lateral band walk, and diagonal band walk

Body Weight Exercises

➢ Squats
➢ Lunges (and reverse lunges)
➢ Pull-ups and chin-ups
➢ Lateral leg raises
➢ Glute bridge and lying hip bridge
➢ Dead bug (lying on floor)
➢ Mountain climbers and spider mountain climbers
➢ Plank and star plank and frozen V-sit
➢ Russian twist
➢ Glute kickback
➢ Superman pose (on floor)
➢ Sit-ups and curls
➢ Push-ups and wall push-ups
➢ Chair dips
➢ Burpees
➢ Standing calf raise

Low-Impact Exercises

➢ Water aerobics and swimming
➢ Pilates
➢ Elliptical workouts
➢ Stationary rowing

- ➤ Cycling: stationary, recumbent, outdoor (flat surfaces)
- ➤ Walking
- ➤ Low-resistance circuit training
- ➤ Yoga
- ➤ Tai Chi
- ➤ Dancing

RESOURCES

CDC: www.cdc.gov

President's Council on Sports, Fitness and Nutrition: www.hhs.gov/fitness

American Heart Association: www.heart.org

Mayo Clinic: www.mayoclinic.org

US Dept. of Health and Human Services: www.hhs.gov

American College of Sports Medicine: www.acsm.org

Medline Plus https://medlineplus.gov/healthrisksofaninactivelifestyle.html

Harvard Health Publishing https://www.health.harvard.edu/staying-healthy/preserve-your-muscle-mass

ABOUT THE AUTHOR

Ms. Laura Sarti is a registered nurse, certified health coach, certified personal trainer and founder of AndiamoFit. Laura holds professional degrees in nursing, sociology, and teaching. Laura is dedicated to helping people overcome obstacles to change. Her ultimate goal is to ease human suffering, the likes of which she has witnessed too much of during her many years working as a nurse. Laura is passionate about supporting people on their healthy living journeys. Laura lives in Maryland. and she enjoys spending time with her friends and family, hiking, traveling, reading, learning how to paint, and exercising her new green thumb!

Made in the USA
Coppell, TX
27 November 2022

87212397R10059